Mediterranean Diet Lifestyle

For who want to try out the Mediterranean Diet

Sasha Merianelli

All rights reserved. Copyright 2021.

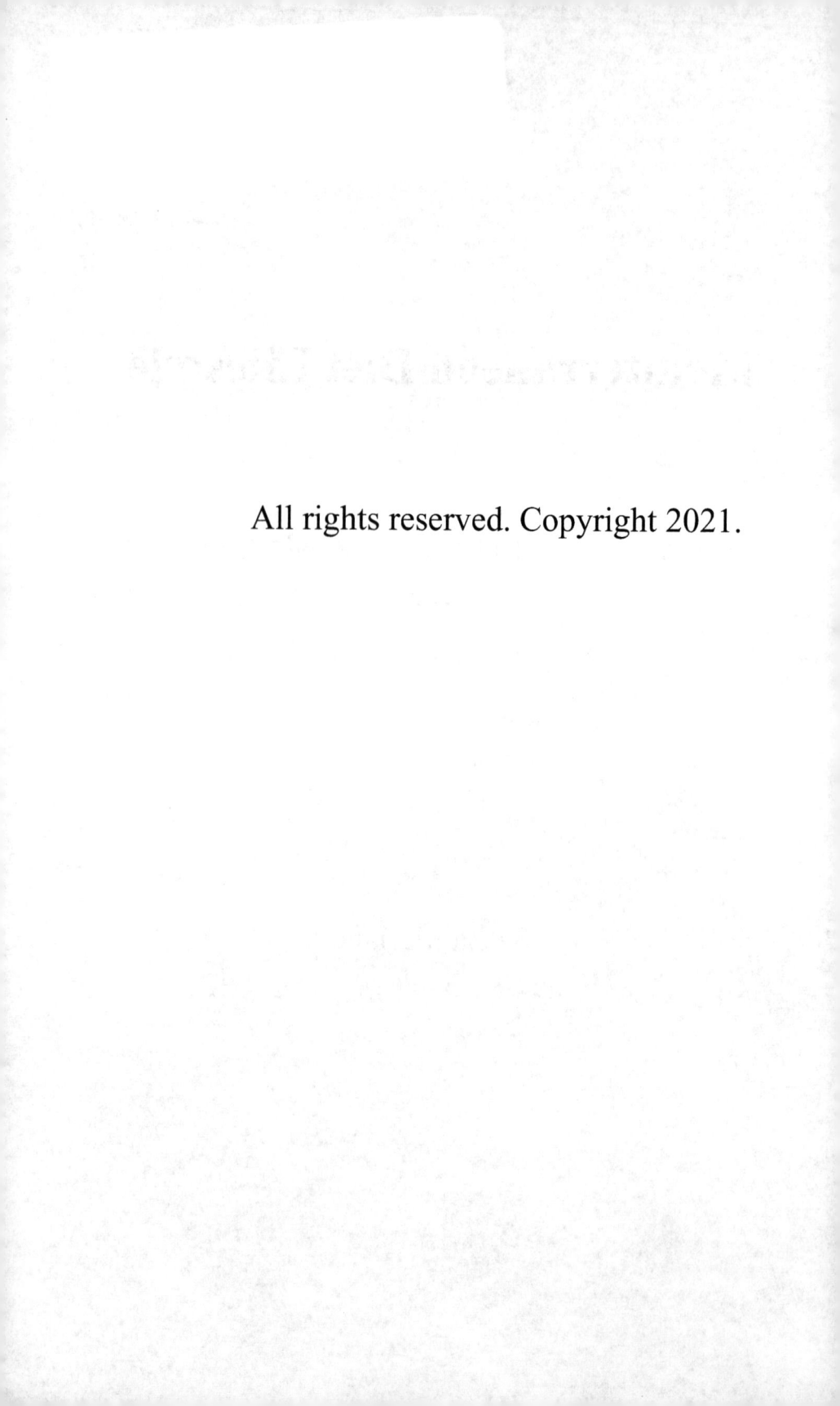

Table of Contents

Grana Padano Risotto 1
Turkey and Bell Pepper Tortiglioni 4
Carrot Risoni 7
Roasted Butternut Squash and Rice 10
Pesto Arborio Rice and Veggie Bowls 13
Rice and Bean Stuffed Zucchini 16
Chard and Mushroom Risotto 19
Cheesy Tomato Linguine 22
Beef and Bean Stuffed Pasta Shells 25
Caprese Fusilli 28
Chicken and Spaghetti Ragù Bolognese 31
Parmesan Squash Linguine 34
Red Bean Curry 36
Stuffed Portobello Mushrooms with Spinach 39
Chickpea Lettuce Wraps with Celery 42
Zoodles with Walnut Pesto 45
Cheesy Sweet Potato Burgers 48
Eggplant and Zucchini Gratin 51
Veggie-Stuffed Portabello Mushrooms 54
Stir-Fried Eggplant 57
Honey-Glazed Baby Carrots 60
Quick Steamed Broccoli 63
Garlic-Butter Asparagus with Parmesan 66
Ratatouille 69

Mushroom and Potato Teriyaki ....

Peanut and Coconut Stuffed Eggplants ....

Cauliflower with Sweet Potato ....

Potato Curry ....

Mushroom, Potato, and Green Bean Mix ....

Mushroom Tacos ....

Lentils and Eggplant Curry ....

Sweet Potato and Tomato Curry ....

Veggie Chili ....

Cabbage Stuffed Acorn Squash ....

Creamy Potato Curry ....

Mushroom and Spinach Stuffed Peppers ....

Black Bean and Corn Tortilla Bowls ....

Cauliflower and Broccoli Bowls ....

Radish and Cabbage Congee 1

Potato and Broccoli Medley 1

Alphabetical Index 1

Grana Padano Risotto

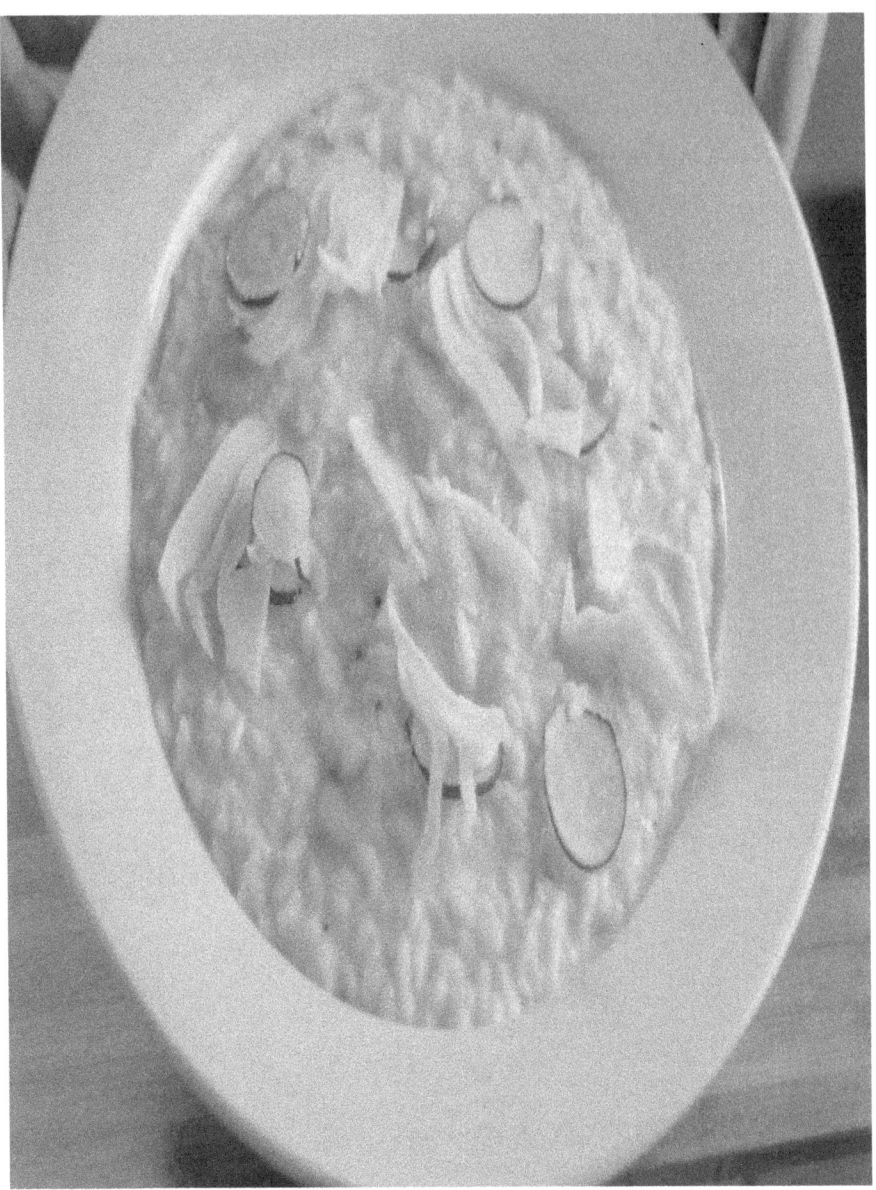

Prep time:
10 minutes | Cook time: 23 minutes | Serves 6

Ingredients

1 tablespoon olive oil

1 white onion, chopped

2 cups Carnaroli rice, rinsed

¼ cup dry white wine

4 cups chicken stock

1 teaspoon salt

½ teaspoon ground white pepper

2 tablespoons Grana padano cheese, grated

¼ tablespoon Grana padano cheese, flakes

Direction

1. Warm oil on Sauté. Stir-fry onion for 3 minutes until soft and translucent. Add rice and cook for 5 minutes stirring occasionally.

2. Pour wine into the pot to deglaze, scrape away any browned bits of food from the pan.

3. Stir in stock, pepper, and salt to the pot. Seal the lid, press Rice and cook on High Pressure for 15 minutes. Release the pressure quickly.

4. Sprinkle with grated Parmesan cheese and stir well. Top with flaked cheese for garnish before serving.

Per Serving

Calories: 307 | fat: 6.0g | protein: 8.2g | carbs: 53.2g | fiber: 2.1g | sodium: 945mg

Turkey and Bell Pepper Tortiglioni

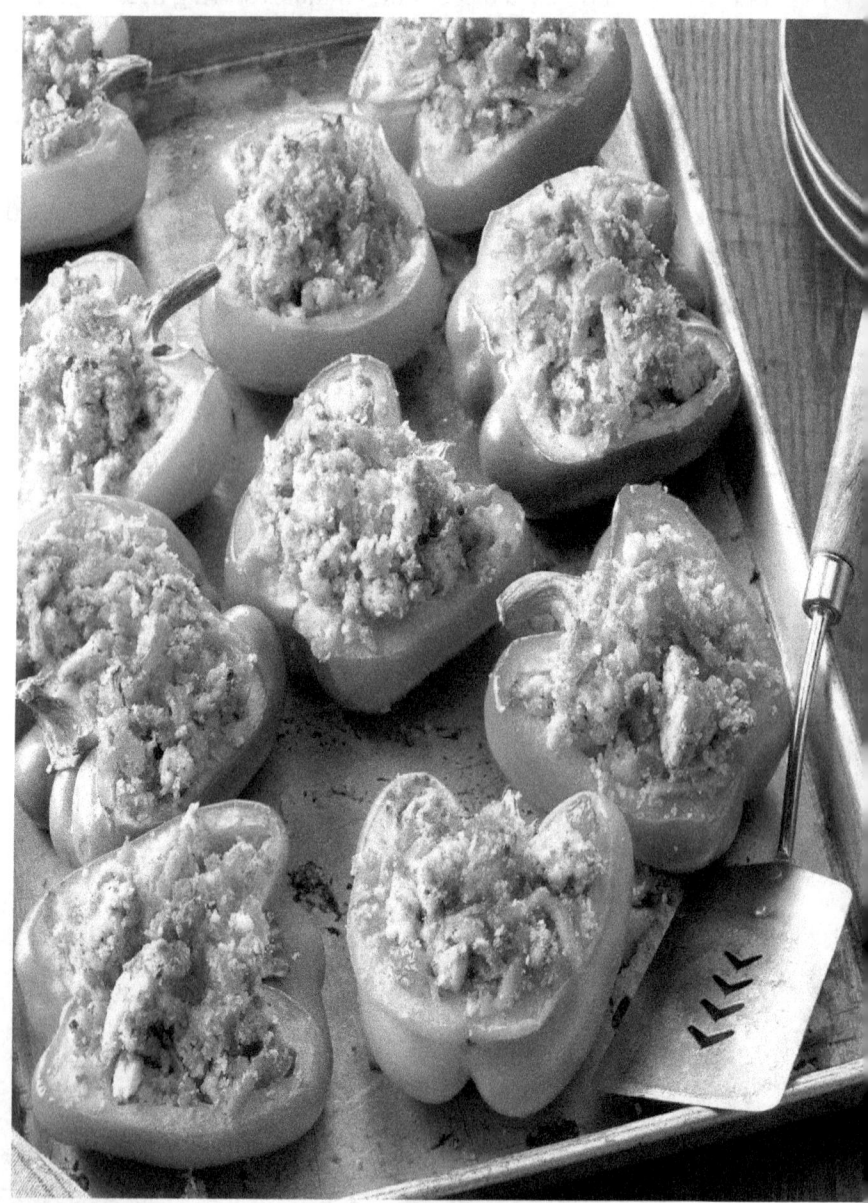

Prep time:
20 minutes | Cook time: 10 minutes | Serves 6

Ingredients

2 teaspoons chili powder

1 teaspoon salt

1 teaspoon cumin

1 teaspoon onion powder

1 teaspoon garlic powder

½ teaspoon thyme

1½ pounds (680 g) turkey breast, cut into strips

1 tablespoon olive oil

1 red onion, cut into wedges

4 garlic cloves, minced

3 cups chicken broth

1 cup salsa

1 pound (454 g) tortiglioni

1 red bell pepper, chopped diagonally

1 yellow bell pepper, chopped diagonally

1 green bell pepper, chopped diagonally

1 cup shredded Gouda cheese

½ cup sour cream

½ cup chopped parsley

Direction

1. In a bowl, mix chili powder, cumin, garlic powder, onion powder, s[alt] and oregano. Reserve 1 teaspoon of seasoning. Coat turkey with remaining seasoning.
2. Warm oil on Sauté. Add turkey strips and sauté for 4 to 5 minutes u[ntil] browned. Place the turkey in a bowl. Sauté the onion and garlic fo[r a] minute in the cooker until soft. Press Cancel.
3. Mix in salsa, broth, and scrape the bottom of any brown bits. Into broth mixture, stir in tortiglioni pasta and cover with bell peppers a[nd] chicken.
4. Seal the lid and cook for 5 minutes on High Pressure. Do a qu[ick] Pressure release.
5. Open the lid and sprinkle with shredded gouda cheese and reserv[ed] seasoning, and stir well. Divide into plates and top with sour cream. A[dd] parsley for garnishing and serve.

Per Serving

Calories: 646 | fat: 21.7g | protein: 41.1g | carbs: 72.9g | fiber: 11.1g | sodiu[m:] 1331mg

Carrot Risoni

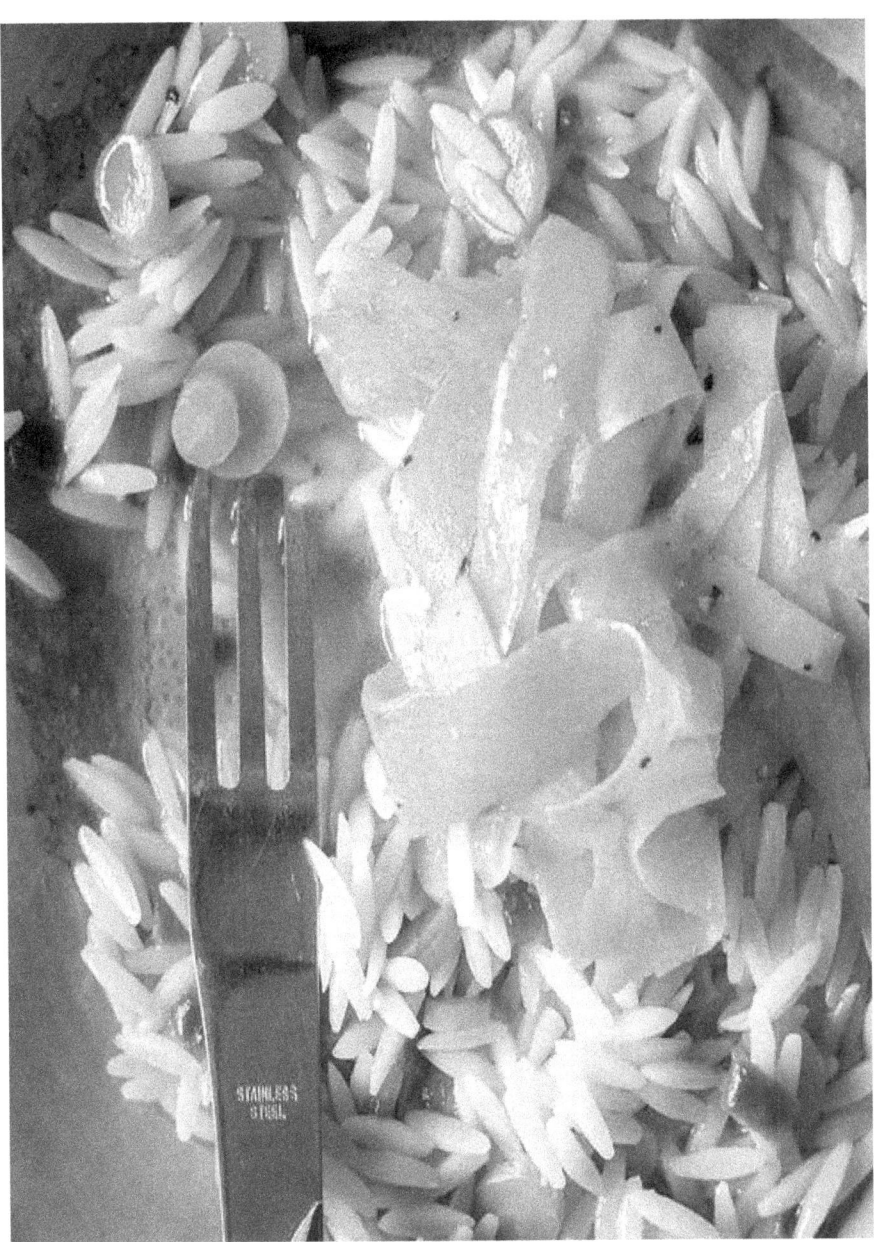

Prep time:
5 minutes | Cook time: 11 minutes | Serves 6

Ingredients

1 cup orzo, rinsed

2 cups water

2 carrots, cut into sticks

1 large onion, chopped

2 tablespoons olive oil

Salt, to taste

Fresh cilantro, chopped, for garnish

Direction

1. Heat oil on Sauté. Add onion and carrots and stir-fry for about 10 minutes until tender and crispy. Remove to a plate and set aside. Add water, salt and orzo in the instant pot.
2. Seal the lid and cook on High Pressure for 1 minute. Do a quick release. Fluff the cooked orzo with a fork. Transfer to a serving plate and top with the carrots and onion. Serve scattered with cilantro.

Per Serving

Calories: 121 | fat: 4.9g | protein: 1.7g | carbs: 18.1g | fiber: 2.9g | sodium: 17mg

Roasted Butternut Squash and Rice

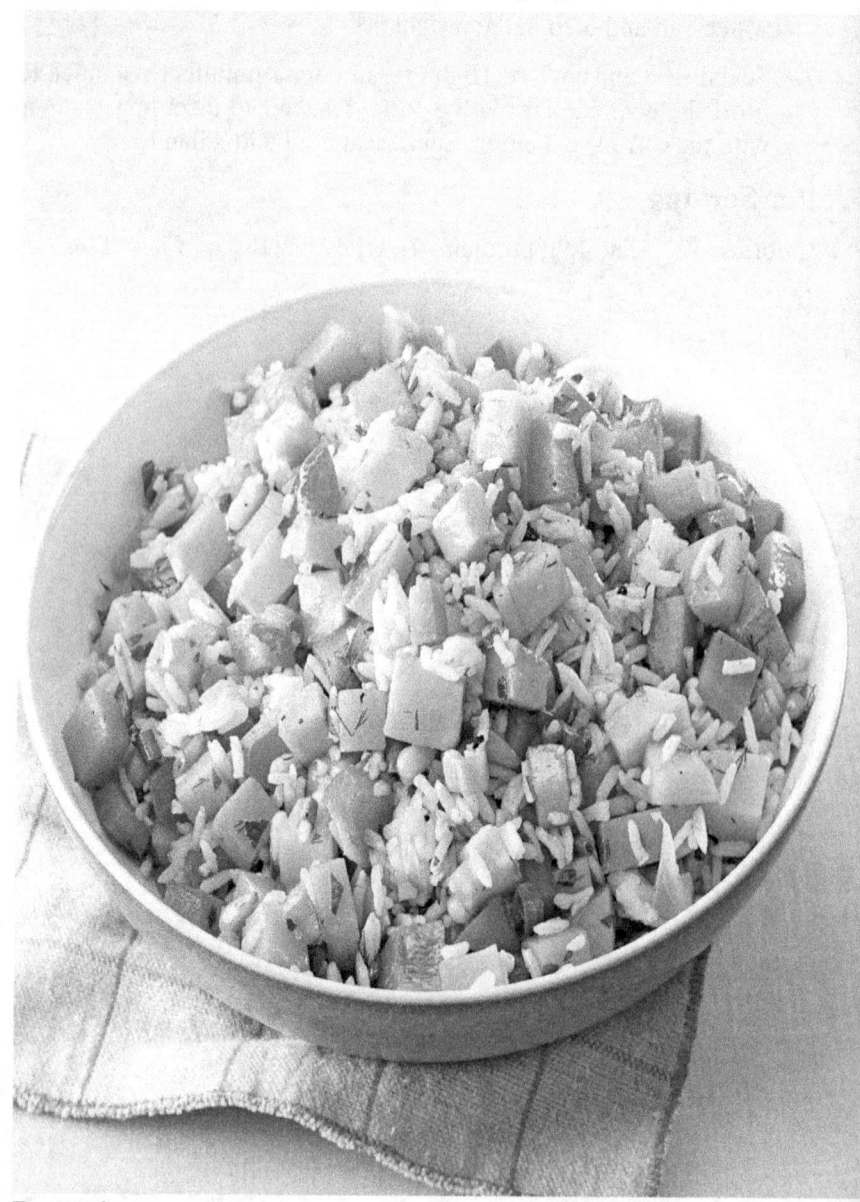

Prep time:

15 minutes | Cook time: 15 minutes | Serves 4

Ingredients

½ cup water

2 cups vegetable broth

1 small butternut squash, peeled and sliced

2 tablespoons olive oil, divided

1 teaspoon salt

1 teaspoon freshly ground black pepper

1 cup feta cheese, cubed

1 tablespoon coconut aminos

2 teaspoons arrowroot starch

1 cup jasmine rice, cooked

Direction

1. Pour the rice and broth in the pot and stir to combine. In a bowl, t butternut squash with 1 tablespoon of olive oil and season with salt black pepper.

2. In another bowl, mix the remaining olive oil, water and coconut amin Toss feta in the mixture, add the arrowroot starch, and toss again combine well. Transfer to a greased baking dish.

3. Lay a trivet over the rice and place the baking dish on the trivet. Seal lid and cook on High for 15 minutes. Do a quick pressure release. Fl the rice with a fork and serve with squash and feta.

Per Serving

Calories: 258 | fat: 14.9g | protein: 7.8g | carbs: 23.2g | fiber: 1.2g | sodiu 1180mg

Pesto Arborio Rice and Veggie Bowls

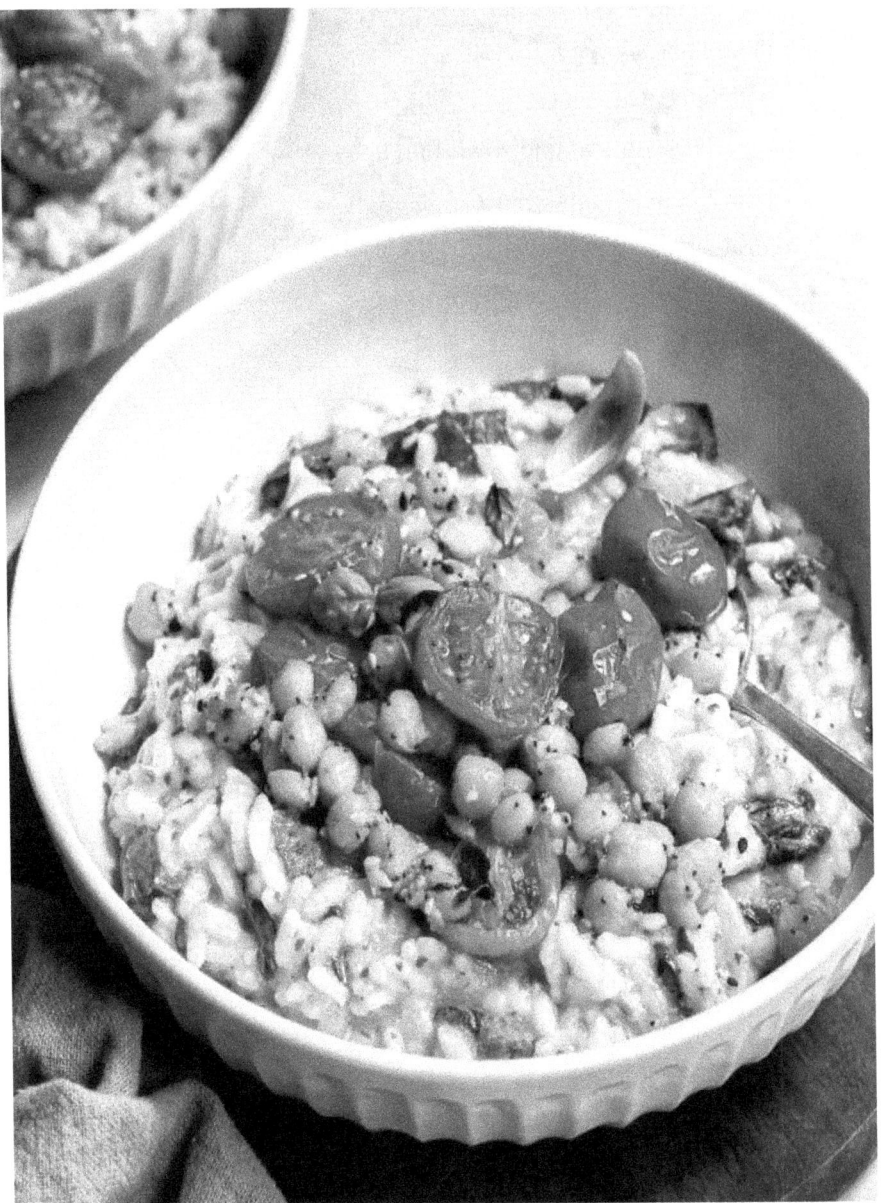

Prep time:
10 minutes | Cook time: 1 minute | Serves 2

Ingredients

1 cup arborio rice, rinsed and drained

2 cups vegetable broth

Salt and black pepper to taste

1 potato, peeled, cubed

1 head broccoli, cut into small florets

1 bunch baby carrots, peeled

¼ cabbage, chopped

2 eggs

¼ cup pesto sauce

Lemon wedges, for serving

Direction

1. In the pot, mix broth, pepper, rice and salt. Set trivet to the inner pot on top of rice and add a steamer basket to the top of the trivet. Mix carrots, potato, eggs and broccoli in the steamer basket. Add pepper and salt for seasoning.
2. Seal the lid and cook for 1 minute on High Pressure. Quick release the pressure.
3. Take away the trivet and steamer basket from the pot. Set the eggs in a bowl of ice water. Then peel and halve the eggs. Use a fork to fluff rice. Adjust the seasonings.
4. In two bowls, equally divide rice, broccoli, eggs, carrots, sweet potatoes, and a dollop of pesto. Serve alongside a lemon wedge.

Per Serving

Calories: 858 | fat: 24.4g | protein: 26.4g | carbs: 136.2g | fiber: 14.1g | sodium: 985mg

Rice and Bean Stuffed Zucchini

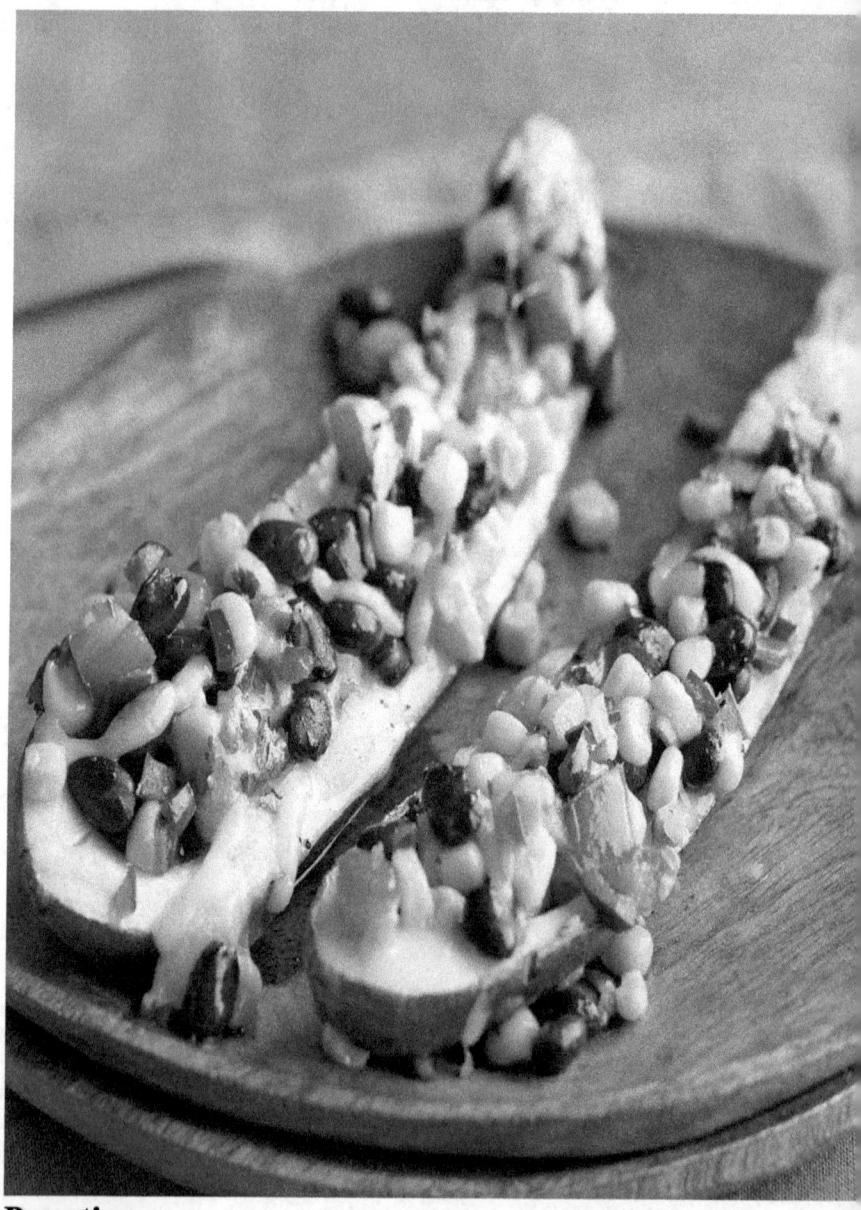

Prep time:
10 minutes | Cook time: 15 minutes | Serves 4

Ingredients

2 small zucchinis, halved lengthwise

½ cup cooked rice

½ cup canned white beans, drained and rinsed

½ cup chopped tomatoes

½ cup chopped toasted cashew nuts

½ cup grated Parmesan cheese

1 tablespoon olive oil

½ teaspoon salt

½ teaspoon freshly ground black pepper

Direction

1. Pour 1 cup of water in the instant pot and insert a trivet. Scoop out pulp of zucchini and chop roughly.
2. In a bowl, mix the zucchini pulp, rice, tomatoes, cashew nuts, ¼ cup Parmesan, olive oil, salt, and black pepper. Fill the zucchini boats with the mixture, and arrange the stuffed boats in a single layer on the trivet. Seal the lid and cook for 15 minutes on Steam on High. Do a quick release and serve.

Per Serving

Calories: 239 | fat: 14.7g | protein: 9.4g | carbs: 19.0g | fiber: 2.6g | sodium 570mg

Chard and Mushroom Risotto

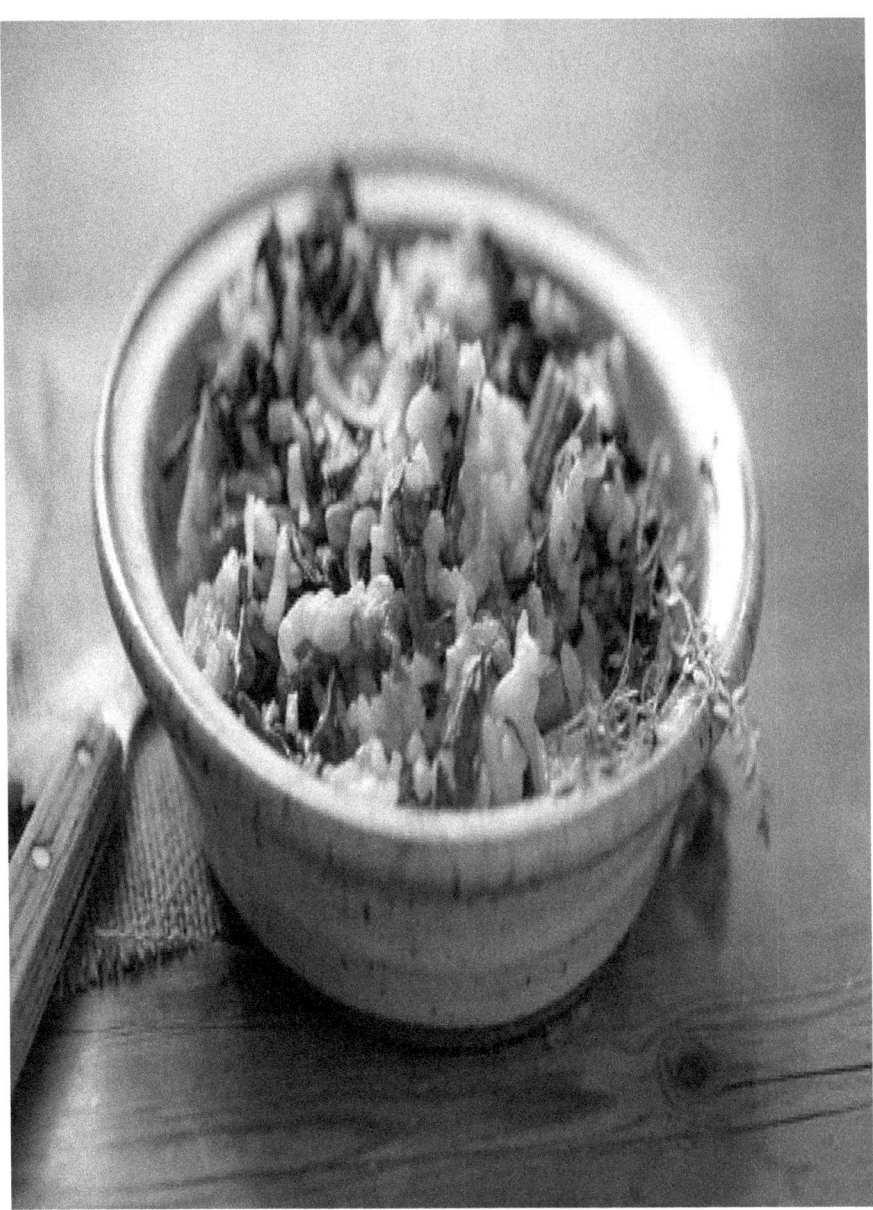

Prep time:
15 minutes | Cook time: 20 minutes | Serves 4

Ingredients

3 tablespoons olive oil

1 onion, chopped

2 Swiss chard, stemmed and chopped

1 cup risotto rice

⅓ cup white wine

3 cups vegetable stock

½ teaspoon salt

½ cup mushrooms

4 tablespoons pumpkin seeds, toasted

⅓ cup grated Pecorino Romano cheese

Direction

1. Heat oil on Sauté, and cook onion and mushrooms for 5 minutes, stirring, until tender. Add the rice and cook for a minute. Stir in wine and cook for 2 to 3 minutes until almost evaporated.

2. Pour in stock and season with salt. Seal the lid and cook on High Pressure for 10 minutes. Do a quick release. Stir in chard until wilted, mix in cheese to melt, and serve scattered with pumpkin seeds.

Per Serving

Calories: 420 | fat: 17.7g | protein: 11.8g | carbs: 54.9g | fiber: 4.9g | sodium: 927mg

Cheesy Tomato Linguine

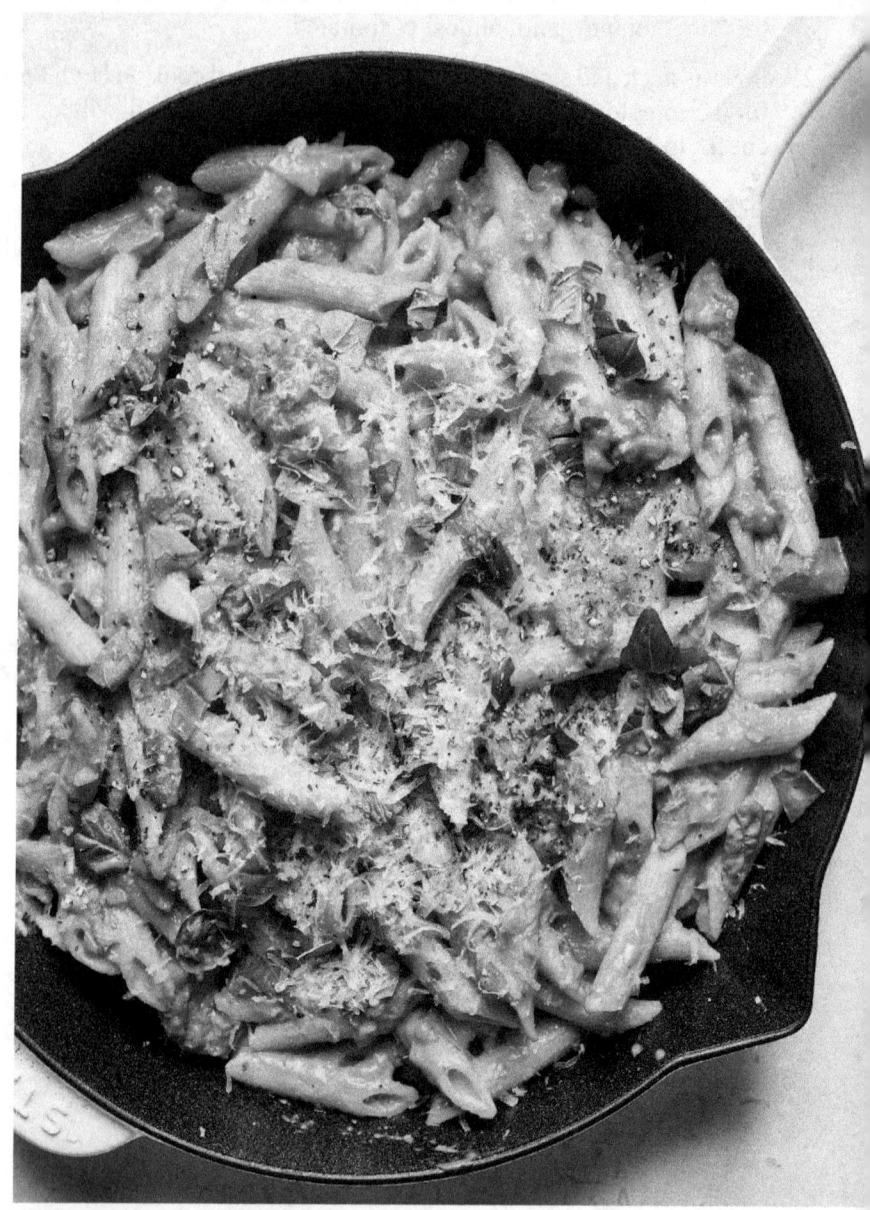

Prep time:

15 minutes | Cook time: 11 minutes | Serves 4

Ingredients

2 tablespoons olive oil

1 small onion, diced

2 garlic cloves, minced

1 cup cherry tomatoes, halved

1½ cups vegetable stock

¼ cup julienned basil leaves

1 teaspoon salt

½ teaspoon ground black pepper

¼ teaspoon red chili flakes

1 pound (454 g) Linguine noodles, halved

Fresh basil leaves for garnish

½ cup Parmigiano-Reggiano cheese, grated

Direction

1. Warm oil on Sauté. Add onion and Sauté for 2 minutes until soft. Ν garlic and tomatoes and sauté for 4 minutes. To the pot, add vegeta stock, salt, julienned basil, red chili flakes and pepper.

2. Add linguine to the tomato mixture until covered. Seal the lid and cc on High Pressure for 5 minutes.

3. Naturally release the pressure for 5 minutes. Stir the mixture to ensur is broken down.

4. Divide into plates. Top with basil and Parmigiano-Reggiano cheese a serve.

Per Serving

Calories: 311 | fat: 11.3g | protein: 10.3g | carbs: 42.1g | fiber: 1.9g | sodiu 1210mg

Beef and Bean Stuffed Pasta Shells

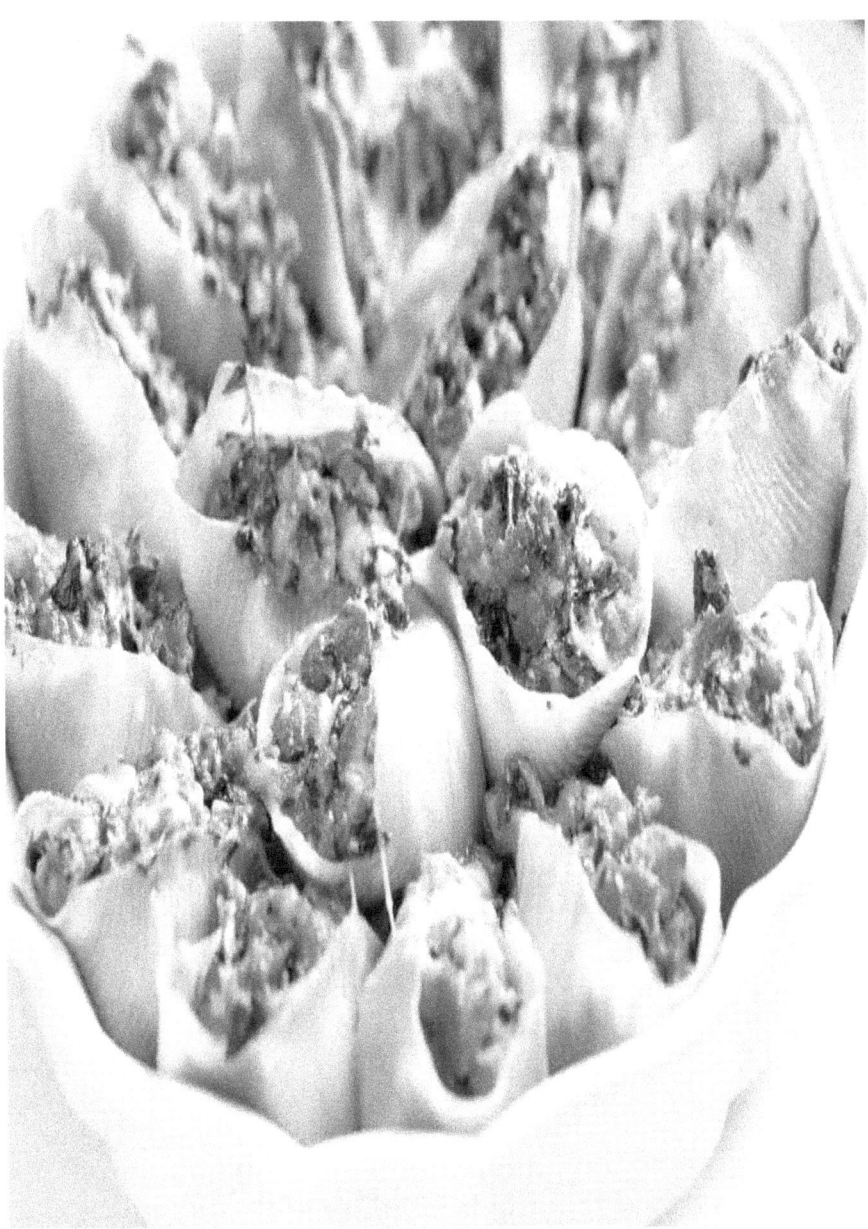

Prep time:
15 minutes | Cook time: 17 minutes | Serves 4

Ingredients

2 tablespoons olive oil

1 pound (454 g) ground beef

1 pound (454 g) pasta shells

2 cups water

15 ounces (425 g) tomato sauce

1 (15-ounce / 425-g) can black beans, drained and rinsed

15 ounces (425 g) canned corn, drained (or 2 cups frozen corn)

10 ounces (283 g) red enchilada sauce

4 ounces (113 g) diced green chiles

1 cup shredded Mozzarella cheese

Salt and ground black pepper to taste

Additional cheese for topping

Finely chopped parsley for garnish

Direction

1. Heat oil on Sauté. Add ground beef and cook for 7 minutes until it starts to brown.

2. Mix in pasta, tomato sauce, enchilada sauce, black beans, water, corn, and green chiles and stir to coat well. Add more water if desired.

3. Seal the lid and cook on High Pressure for 10 minutes. Do a quick Pressure release. Into the pasta mixture, mix in Mozzarella cheese until melted; add black pepper and salt. Garnish with parsley to serve.

Per Serving

Calories: 1006 | fat: 30.0g | protein: 53.3g | carbs: 138.9g | fiber: 24.4g | sodium: 1139mg

Caprese Fusilli

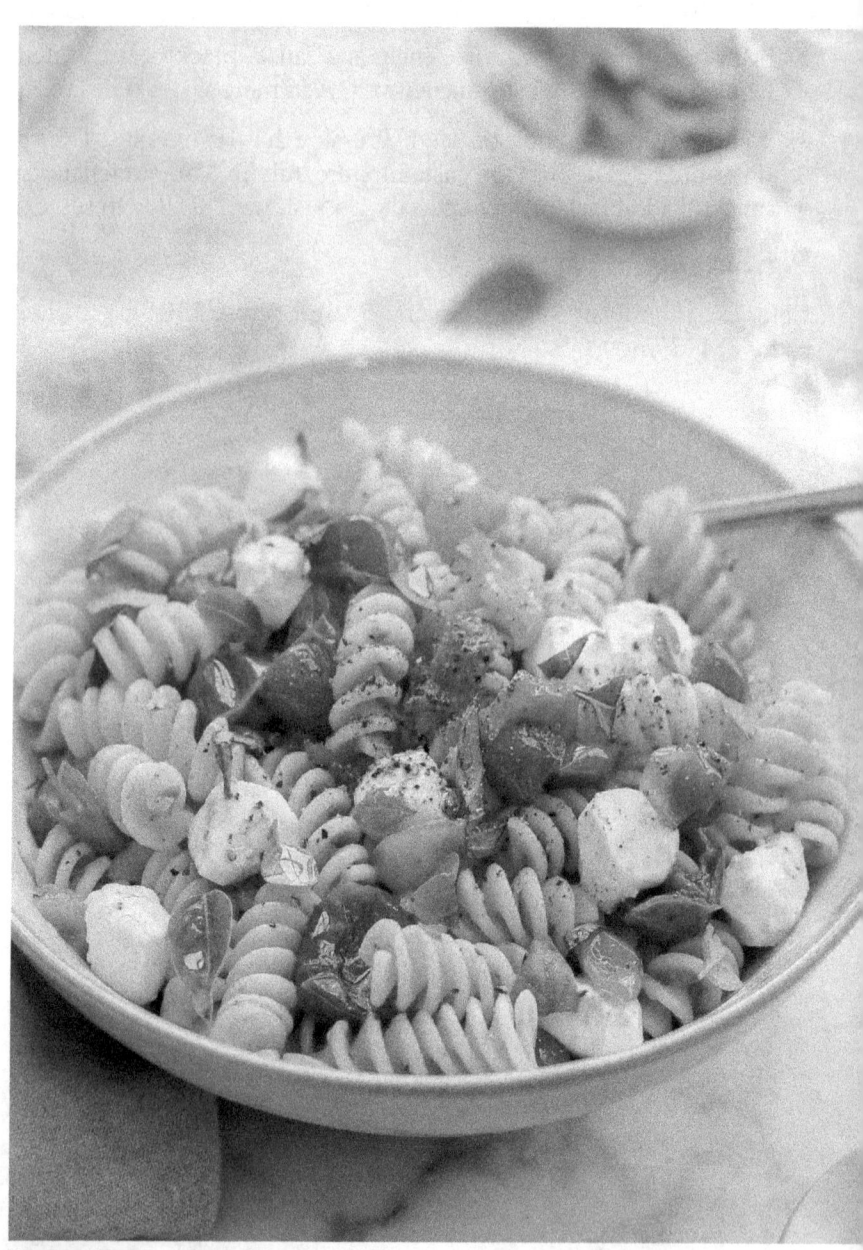

Prep time:
15 minutes | Cook time: 7 minutes | Serves 3

Ingredients

1 tablespoon olive oil

1 onion, thinly chopped

6 garlic cloves, minced

1 teaspoon red pepper flakes

2½ cups dried fusilli

1 (15-ounce / 425-g) can tomato sauce

1 cup tomatoes, halved

1 cup water

¼ cup basil leaves

1 teaspoon salt

1 cup Ricotta cheese, crumbled

2 tablespoons chopped fresh basil

Direction

1. Warm oil on Sauté. Add red pepper flakes, garlic and onion and cook 3 minutes until soft.

2. Mix in fusilli, tomatoes, half of the basil leaves, water, tomato sauce, and salt. Seal the lid, and cook on High Pressure for 4 minutes. Release pressure quickly.

3. Transfer the pasta to a serving platter and top with the crumbled ricc and remaining chopped basil.

Per Serving

Calories: 589 | fat: 17.7g | protein: 19.5g | carbs: 92.8g | fiber: 13.8g | sodiu 879mg

Chicken and Spaghetti Ragù Bolognese

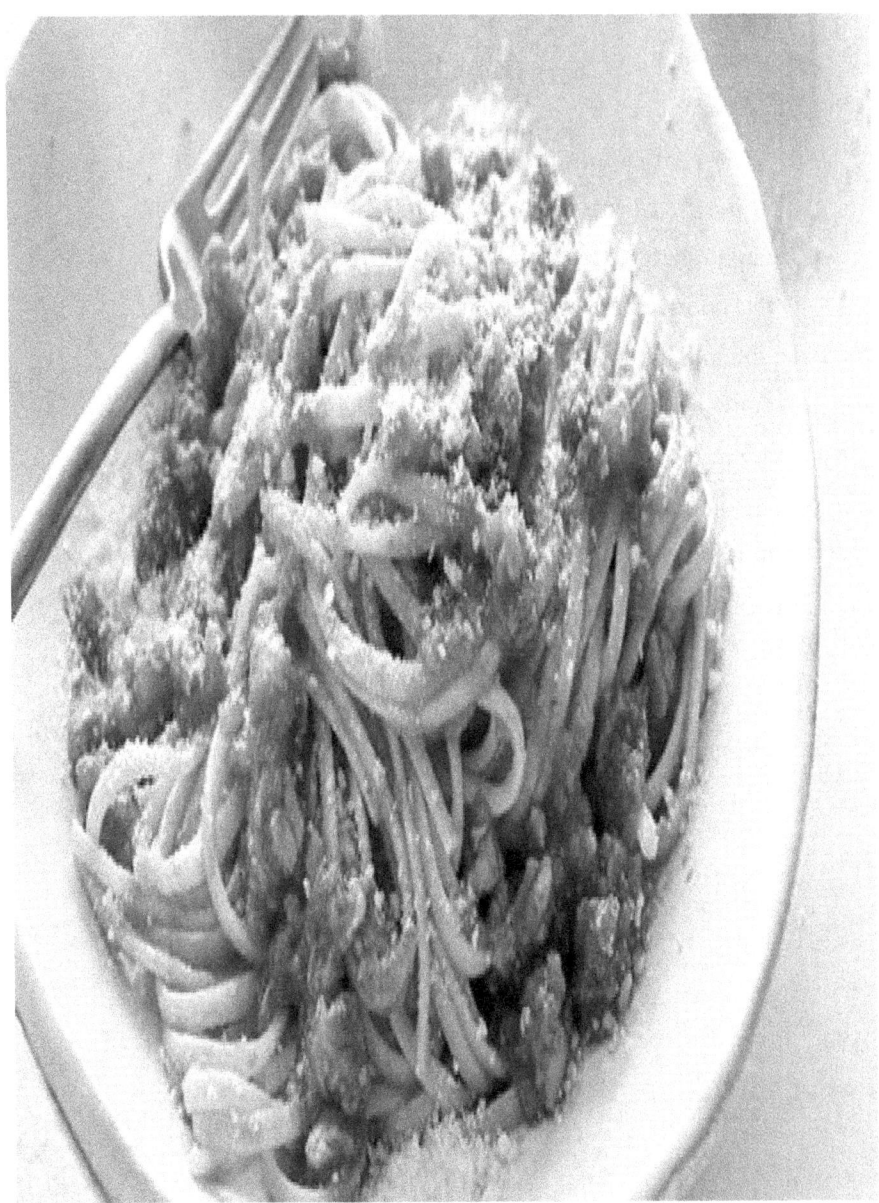

Prep time:
15 minutes | Cook time: 42 minutes | Serves 8

Ingredients

2 tablespoons olive oil

6 ounces (170 g) bacon, cubed

1 onion, minced

1 carrot, minced

1 celery stalk, minced

2 garlic cloves, crushed

¼ cup tomato paste

¼ teaspoon crushed red pepper flakes

1½ pounds (680 g) ground chicken

½ cup white wine

1 cup milk

1 cup chicken broth

Salt, to taste

1 pound (454 g) spaghetti

Direction

1. Warm oil on Sauté. Add bacon and fry for 5 minutes until crispy.

2. Add celery, carrot, garlic and onion and cook for 5 minutes until fragrant. Mix in red pepper flakes and tomato paste, and cook for 2 minutes. Break chicken into small pieces and place in the pot.

3. Cook for 10 minutes, as you stir, until browned. Pour in wine and simmer for 2 minutes. Add chicken broth and milk. Seal the lid and cook for 15 minutes on High Pressure. Release the pressure quickly.

4. Add the spaghetti and stir. Seal the lid, and cook on High Pressure for another 5 minutes.

5. Release the pressure quickly. Check the pasta for doneness. Taste, adjust the seasoning and serve hot.

Per Serving

Calories: 477 | fat: 20.6g | protein: 28.1g | carbs: 48.5g | fiber: 5.3g | sodium: 279mg

Parmesan Squash Linguine

Prep time:

15 minutes | Cook time: 5 minutes | Serves 4

Ingredients

1 cup flour

2 teaspoons salt

2 eggs

4 cups water

1 cup seasoned breadcrumbs

½ cup grated Parmesan cheese, plus more for garnish

1 yellow squash, peeled and sliced

1 pound (454 g) linguine

24 ounces (680 g) canned seasoned tomato sauce

2 tablespoons olive oil

1 cup shredded Mozzarella cheese

Minced fresh basil, for garnish

Direction

1. Break the linguine in half. Put it in the pot and add water and half of salt. Seal the lid and cook on High Pressure for 5 minutes. Combine the flour and 1 teaspoon of salt in a bowl. In another bowl, whisk the eggs and 2 tablespoons of water. In a third bowl, mix the breadcrumbs and Mozzarella cheese.

2. Coat each squash slices in the flour. Shake off excess flour, dip in the egg wash, and dredge in the bread crumbs. Set aside. Quickly release the pressure. Remove linguine to a serving bowl and mix in the tomato sauce and sprinkle with fresh basil. Heat oil on Sauté and fry breaded squash until crispy.

3. Serve the squash topped Mozzarella cheese with the linguine on side.

Per Serving

Calories: 857 | fat: 17.0g | protein: 33.2g | carbs: 146.7g | fiber: 18.1g | sodium: 1856mg

Red Bean Curry

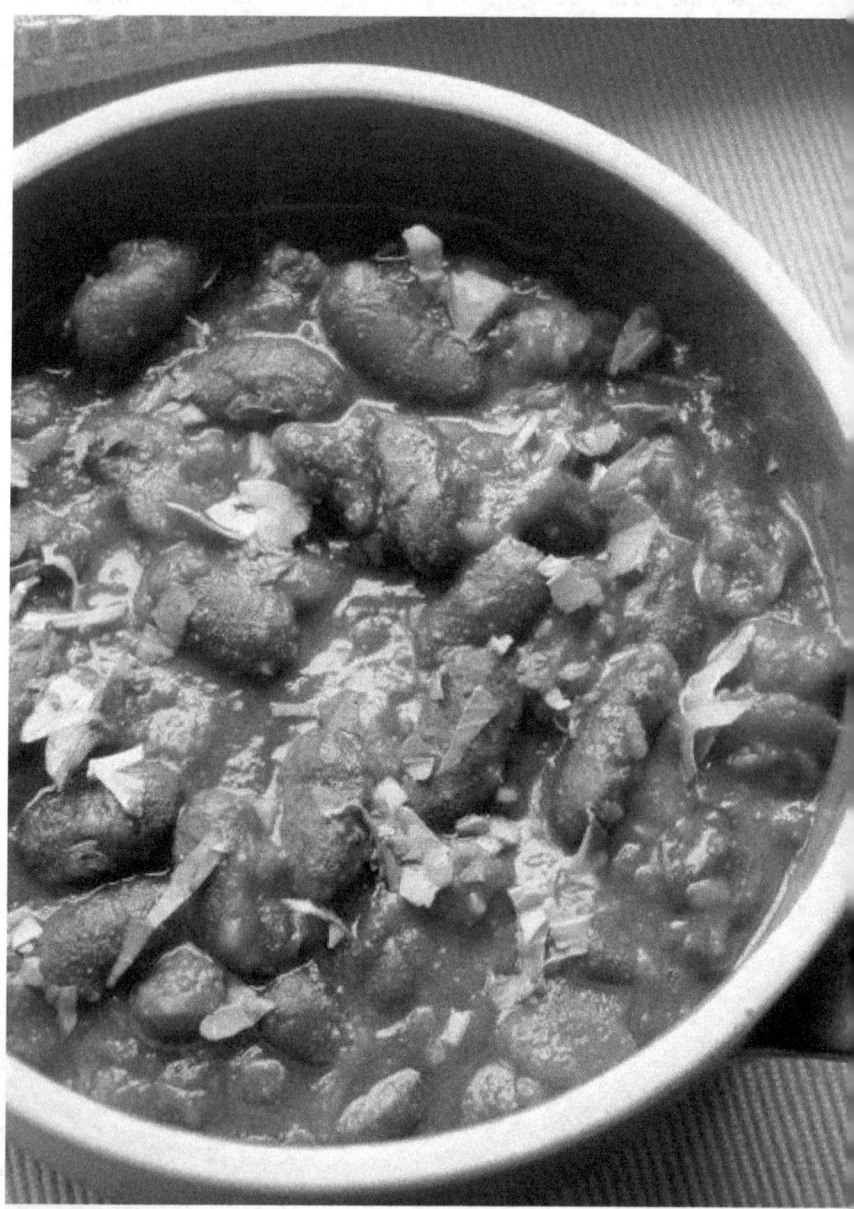

Prep time:

10 minutes | Cook time: 24 minutes | Serves 4

Ingredients

½ cup raw red beans

1½ tablespoons cooking oil

½ cup chopped onions

1 bay leaf

½ tablespoon grated garlic

¼ tablespoon grated ginger

¾ cup water

1 cup fresh tomato purée

½ green chili, finely chopped

¼ teaspoon turmeric

½ teaspoon coriander powder

1 teaspoon chili powder

1 cup chopped baby spinach

Salt, to taste

Boiled white rice or quinoa, for serve

Direction

1. Add the oil and onions to the Instant Pot. Sauté for 5 minutes.
2. Stir in ginger, garlic paste, green chili and bay leaf. Cook for 1 minute then add all the spices.
3. Add the red beans, tomato purée and water to the pot.
4. Cover and secure the lid. Turn its pressure release handle to the sealing position.
5. Cook on the Manual function with High Pressure for 15 minutes.
6. After the beep, do a Natural release for 20 minutes.
7. Stir in spinach and cook for 3 minutes on the Sauté setting.
8. Serve hot with boiled white rice or quinoa.

Per Serving

Calories: 159 | fat: 5.6g | protein: 6.8g | carbs: 22.5g | fiber: 5.5g | sodium 182mg

Stuffed Portobello Mushrooms with Spinach

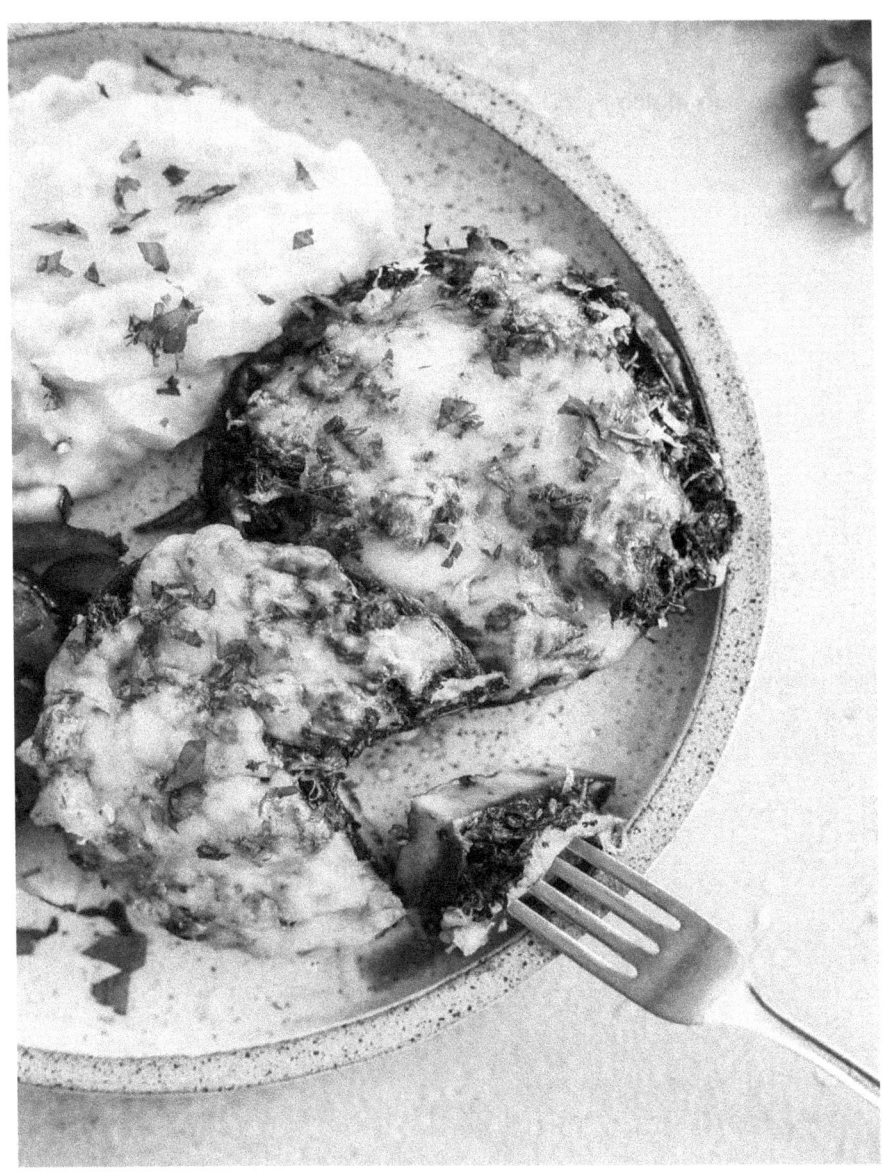

Prep time:
5 minutes | Cook time: 20 minutes | Serves 4

Ingredients

8 large portobello mushrooms, stems removed

3 teaspoons extra-virgin olive oil, divided

1 medium red bell pepper, diced

4 cups fresh spinach

¼ cup crumbled feta cheese

Direction

1. Preheat the oven to 450°F (235°C).
2. Using a spoon to scoop out the gills of the mushrooms and discard them. Brush the mushrooms with 2 teaspoons of olive oil.
3. Arrange the mushrooms (cap-side down) on a baking sheet. Roast in the preheated oven for 20 minutes.
4. Meantime, in a medium skillet, heat the remaining olive oil over medium heat until it shimmers.
5. Add the bell pepper and spinach and sauté for 8 to 10 minutes, stirring occasionally, or until the spinach is wilted.
6. Remove the mushrooms from the oven to a paper towel-lined plate. Using a spoon to stuff each mushroom with the bell pepper and spinach mixture. Scatter the feta cheese all over.
7. Serve immediately.

Per Serving (2 mushrooms)

Calories: 115 | fat: 5.9g | protein: 7.2g | carbs: 11.5g | fiber: 4.0g | sodium: 125mg

Chickpea Lettuce Wraps with Celery

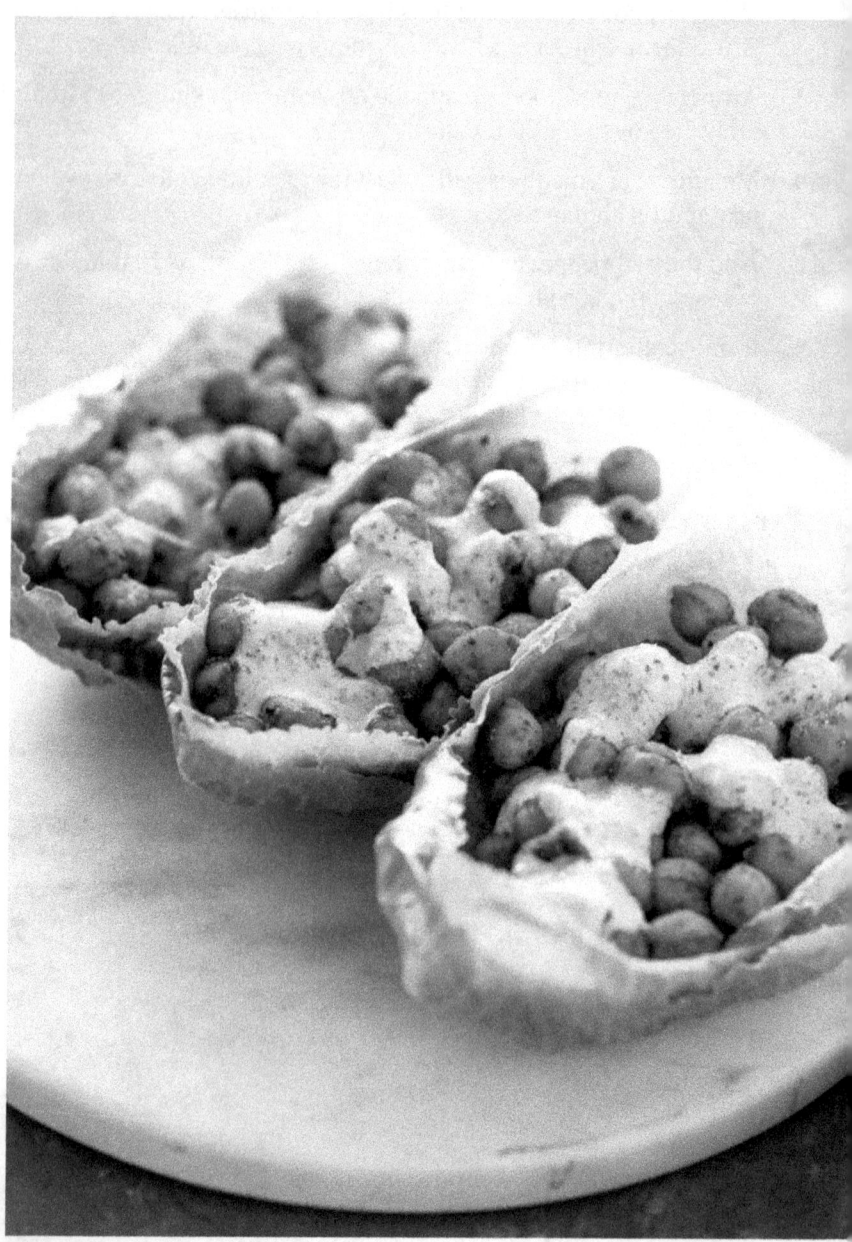

Prep time:
10 minutes | Cook time: 0 minutes | Serves 4

Ingredients

1 (15-ounce / 425-g) can low-sodium chickpeas, drained and rinsed

1 celery stalk, thinly sliced

2 tablespoons finely chopped red onion

2 tablespoons unsalted tahini

3 tablespoons honey mustard

1 tablespoon capers, undrained

12 butter lettuce leaves

Direction

1. In a bowl, mash the chickpeas with a potato masher or the back of a fo until mostly smooth.
2. Add the celery, red onion, tahini, honey mustard, and capers to the bo and stir until well incorporated.
3. For each serving, place three overlapping lettuce leaves on a plate a top with ¼ of the mashed chickpea filling, then roll up. Repeat with t remaining lettuce leaves and chickpea mixture.

Per Serving

Calories: 182 | fat: 7.1g | protein: 10.3g | carbs: 19.6g | fiber: 3.0g | sodiur 171mg

Zoodles with Walnut Pesto

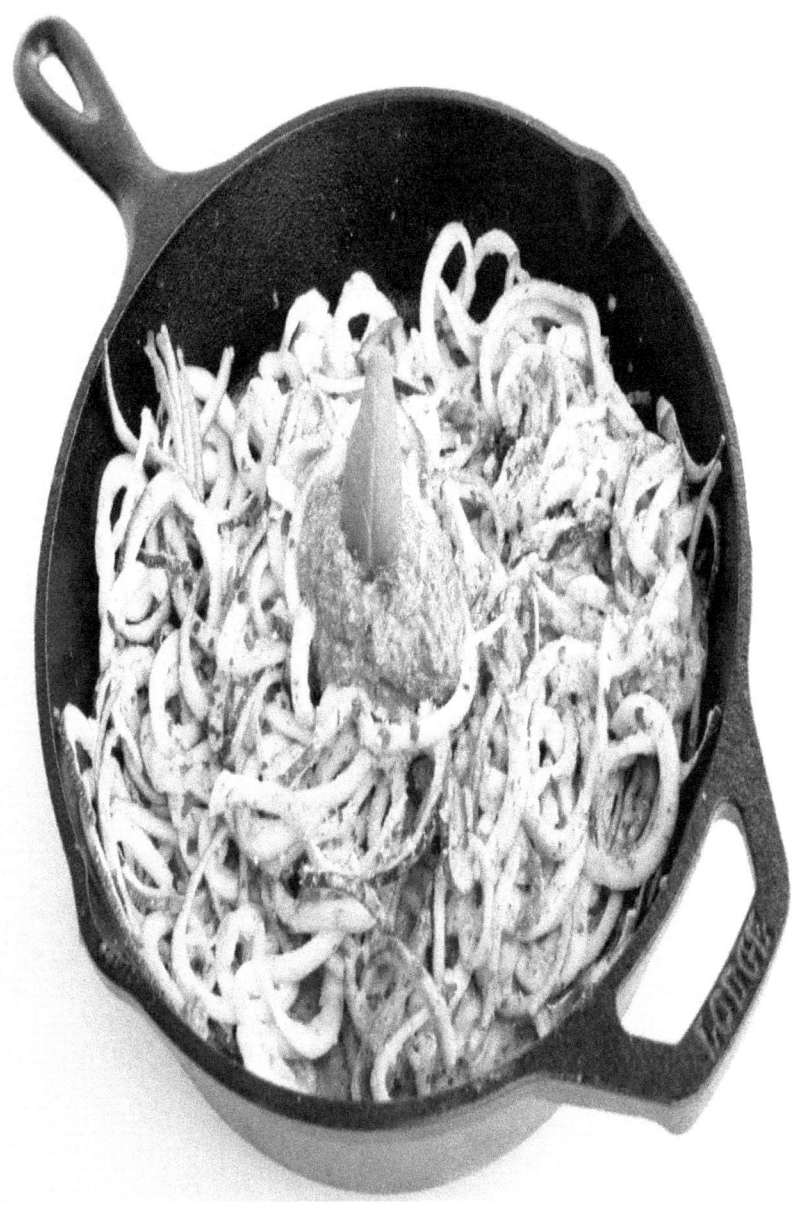

Prep time:
10 minutes | Cook time: 10 minutes | Serves 4

Ingredients

4 medium zucchinis, spiralized

¼ cup extra-virgin olive oil, divided

1 teaspoon minced garlic, divided

½ teaspoon crushed red pepper

¼ teaspoon freshly ground black pepper, divided

¼ teaspoon kosher salt, divided

2 tablespoons grated Parmesan cheese, divided

1 cup packed fresh basil leaves

¾ cup walnut pieces, divided

Direction

1. In a large bowl, stir together the zoodles, 1 tablespoon of the olive oil, ½ teaspoon of the minced garlic, red pepper, ⅛ teaspoon of the black pepper and ⅛ teaspoon of the salt. Set aside.

2. Heat ½ tablespoon of the oil in a large skillet over medium-high heat. Add half of the zoodles to the skillet and cook for 5 minutes, stirring constantly. Transfer the cooked zoodles into a bowl. Repeat with another ½ tablespoon of the oil and the remaining zoodles. When done, add the cooked zoodles to the bowl.

3. Make the pesto: In a food processor, combine the remaining ½ teaspoon of the minced garlic, ⅛ teaspoon of the black pepper and ⅛ teaspoon of the salt, 1 tablespoon of the Parmesan, basil leaves and ¼ cup of the walnuts. Pulse until smooth and then slowly drizzle the remaining 2 tablespoons of the oil into the pesto. Pulse again until well combined.

4. Add the pesto to the zoodles along with the remaining 1 tablespoon of the Parmesan and the remaining ½ cup of the walnuts. Toss to coat well.

5. Serve immediately.

Per Serving

Calories: 166 | fat: 16.0g | protein: 4.0g | carbs: 3.0g | fiber: 2.0g | sodium: 307mg

Cheesy Sweet Potato Burgers

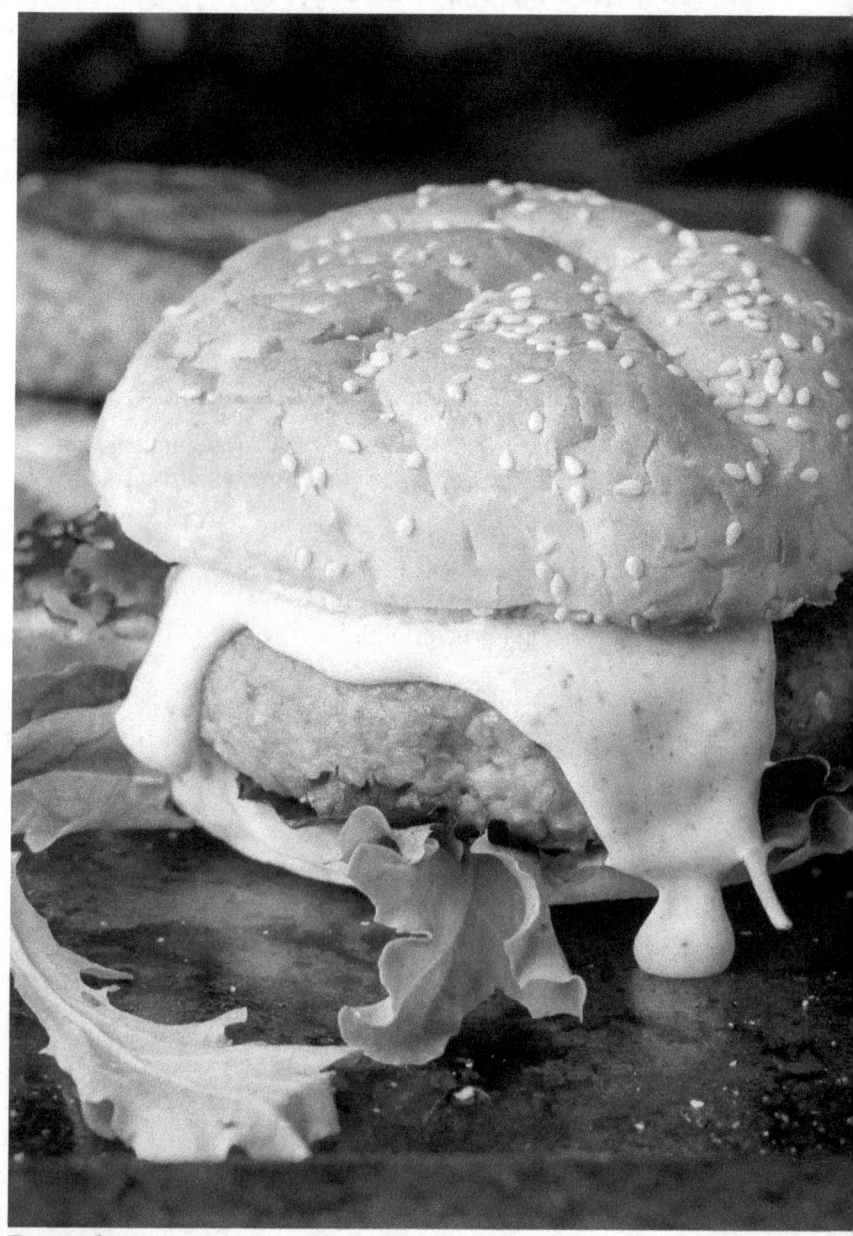

Prep time:

10 minutes | Cook time: 19 to 20 minutes | Serves 4

Ingredients

1 large sweet potato (about 8 ounces / 227 g)

2 tablespoons extra-virgin olive oil, divided

1 cup chopped onion

1 large egg

1 garlic clove

1 cup old-fashioned rolled oats

1 tablespoon dried oregano

1 tablespoon balsamic vinegar

¼ teaspoon kosher salt

½ cup crumbled Gorgonzola cheese

Direction

1. Using a fork, pierce the sweet potato all over and microwave on high 4 to 5 minutes, until softened in the center. Cool slightly before slicing in half.
2. Meanwhile, in a large skillet over medium-high heat, heat 1 tablespoon of the olive oil. Add the onion and sauté for 5 minutes.
3. Spoon the sweet potato flesh out of the skin and put the flesh in a food processor. Add the cooked onion, egg, garlic, oats, oregano, vinegar and salt. Pulse until smooth. Add the cheese and pulse four times to barely combine.
4. Form the mixture into four burgers. Place the burgers on a plate, and press to flatten each to about ¾-inch thick.
5. Wipe out the skillet with a paper towel. Heat the remaining 1 tablespoon of the oil over medium-high heat for about 2 minutes. Add the burgers to the hot oil, then reduce the heat to medium. Cook the burgers for minutes per side.
6. Transfer the burgers to a plate and serve.

Per Serving

Calories: 290 | fat: 12.0g | protein: 12.0g | carbs: 43.0g | fiber: 8.0g | sodium 566mg

Eggplant and Zucchini Gratin

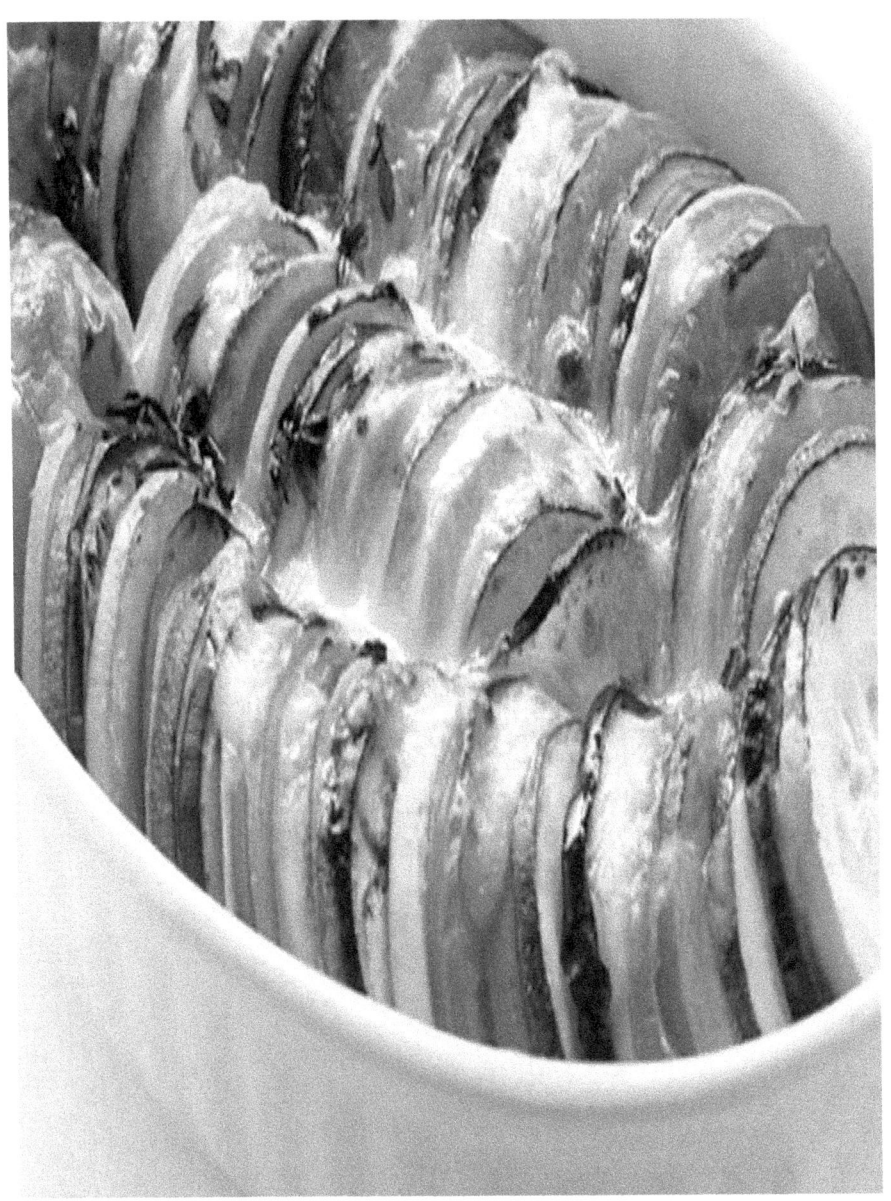

Prep time:
10 minutes | Cook time: 19 minutes | Serves 6

Ingredients

2 large zucchinis, finely chopped

1 large eggplant, finely chopped

¼ teaspoon kosher salt

¼ teaspoon freshly ground black pepper

3 tablespoons extra-virgin olive oil, divided

¾ cup unsweetened almond milk

1 tablespoon all-purpose flour

⅓ cup plus 2 tablespoons grated Parmesan cheese, divided

1 cup chopped tomato

1 cup diced fresh Mozzarella

¼ cup fresh basil leaves

Direction

1. Preheat the oven to 425°F (220°C).
2. In a large bowl, toss together the zucchini, eggplant, salt and pepper.
3. In a large skillet over medium-high heat, heat 1 tablespoon of the oil. Add half of the veggie mixture to the skillet. Stir a few times, then cover and cook for about 4 minutes, stirring occasionally. Pour the cooked veggies into a baking dish. Place the skillet back on the heat, add 1 tablespoon of the oil and repeat with the remaining veggies. Add the veggies to the baking dish.
4. Meanwhile, heat the milk in the microwave for 1 minute. Set aside.
5. Place a medium saucepan over medium heat. Add the remaining 1 tablespoon of the oil and flour to the saucepan. Whisk together until well blended.
6. Slowly pour the warm milk into the saucepan, whisking the entire time. Continue to whisk frequently until the mixture thickens a bit. Add ⅓ cup of the Parmesan cheese and whisk until melted. Pour the cheese sauce over the vegetables in the baking dish and mix well.
7. Fold in the tomatoes and Mozzarella cheese. Roast in the oven for 10 minutes, or until the gratin is almost set and not runny.
8. Top with the fresh basil leaves and the remaining 2 tablespoons of the Parmesan cheese before serving.

Per Serving

Calories: 122 | fat: 5.0g | protein: 10.0g | carbs: 11.0g | fiber: 4.0g | sodium: 364mg

Veggie-Stuffed Portabello Mushrooms

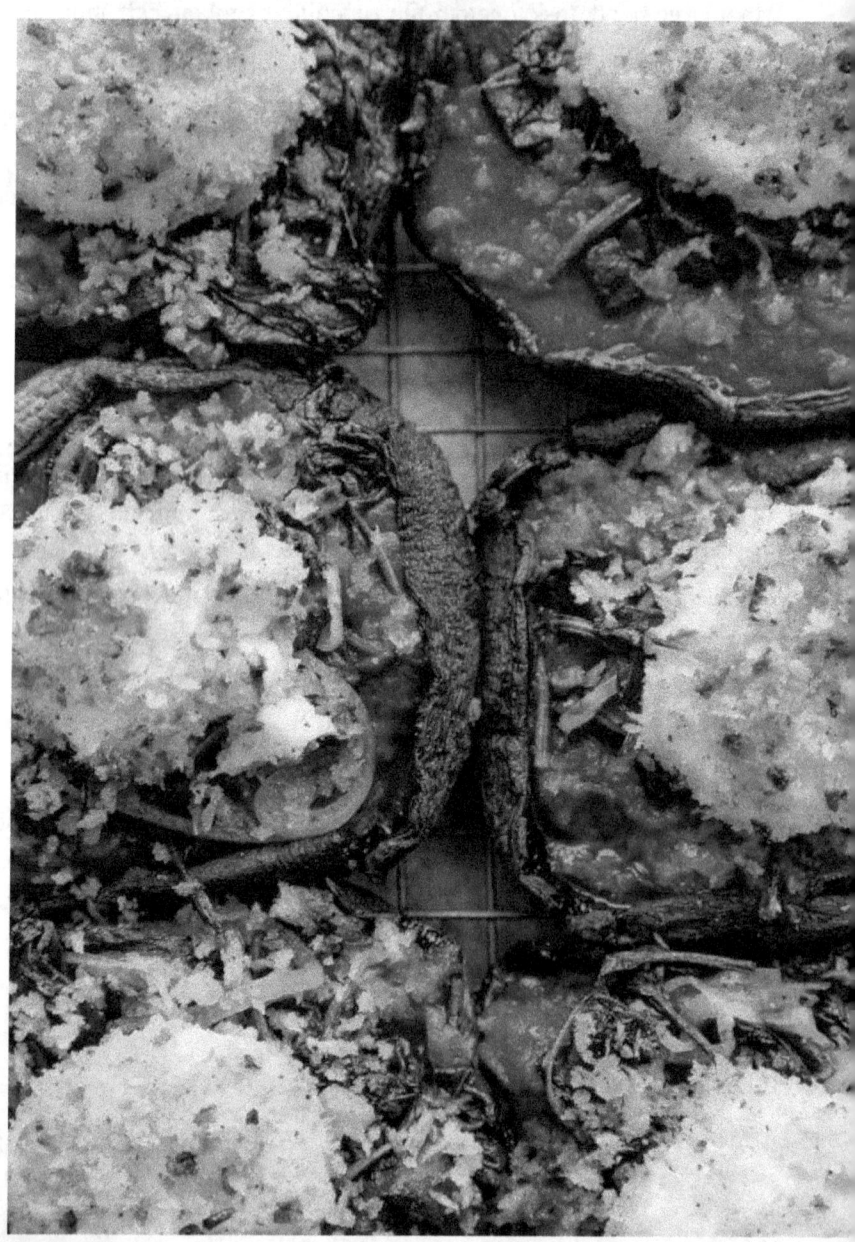

Prep time:

5 minutes | Cook time: 24 to 25 minutes | Serves 6

Ingredients

3 tablespoons extra-virgin olive oil, divided

1 cup diced onion

2 garlic cloves, minced

1 large zucchini, diced

3 cups chopped mushrooms

1 cup chopped tomato

1 teaspoon dried oregano

¼ teaspoon kosher salt

¼ teaspoon crushed red pepper

6 large portabello mushrooms, stems and gills removed

Cooking spray

4 ounces (113 g) fresh Mozzarella cheese, shredded

Direction

1. In a large skillet over medium heat, heat 2 tablespoons of the oil. A the onion and sauté for 4 minutes. Stir in the garlic and sauté for minute.
2. Stir in the zucchini, mushrooms, tomato, oregano, salt and red pepp Cook for 10 minutes, stirring constantly. Remove from the heat.
3. Meanwhile, heat a grill pan over medium-high heat.
4. Brush the remaining 1 tablespoon of the oil over the portabe mushroom caps. Place the mushrooms, bottom-side down, on the gr pan. Cover with a sheet of aluminum foil sprayed with nonstick cooki spray. Cook for 5 minutes.
5. Flip the mushroom caps over, and spoon about ½ cup of the cook vegetable mixture into each cap. Top each with about 2½ tablespoons the Mozzarella.
6. Cover and grill for 4 to 5 minutes, or until the cheese is melted.
7. Using a spatula, transfer the portabello mushrooms to a plate. Let co for about 5 minutes before serving.

Per Serving

Calories: 111 | fat: 4.0g | protein: 11.0g | carbs: 11.0g | fiber: 4.0g | sodiur 314mg

Stir-Fried Eggplant

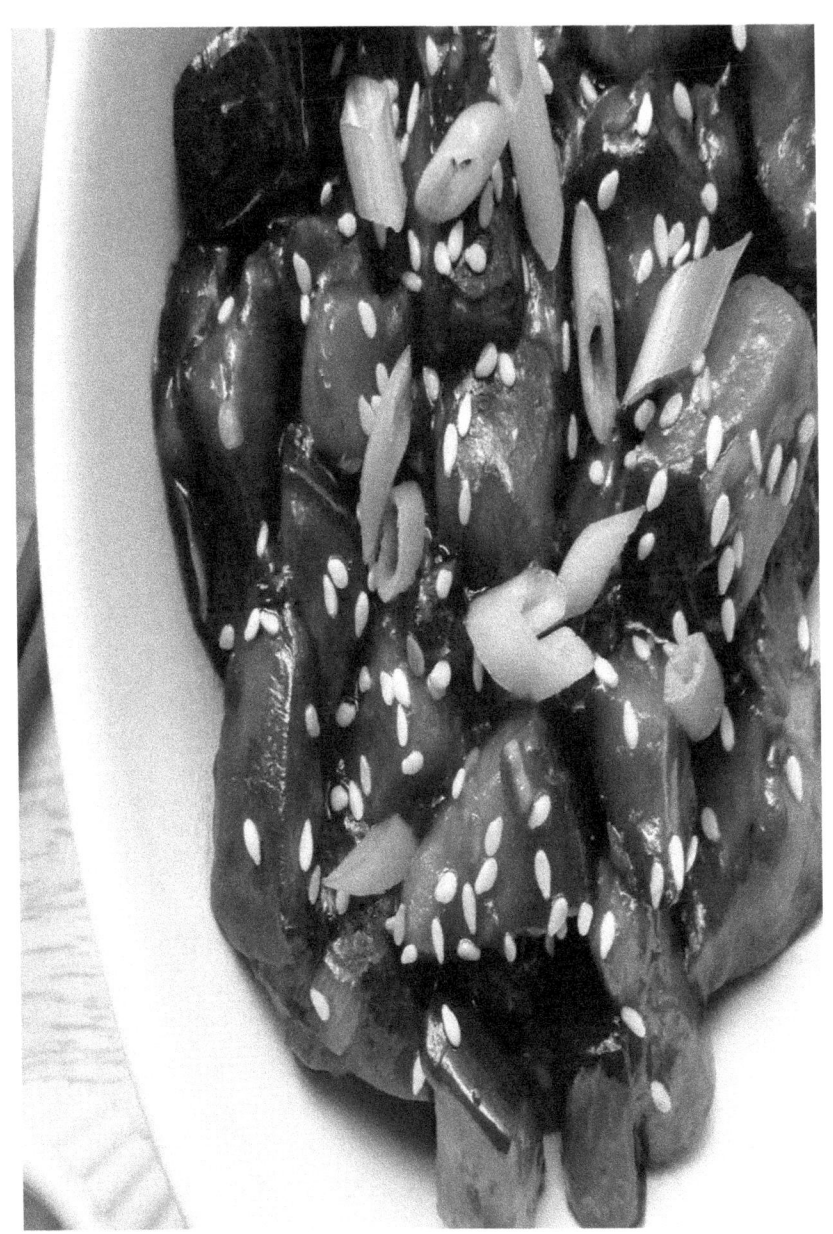

Prep time:
25 minutes | Cook time: 15 minutes | Serves 2

Ingredients

1 cup water, plus more as needed

½ cup chopped red onion

1 tablespoon finely chopped garlic

1 tablespoon dried Italian herb seasoning

1 teaspoon ground cumin

1 small eggplant (about 8 ounces / 227 g), peeled and cut into ½-inch cube

1 medium carrot, sliced

2 cups green beans, cut into 1-inch pieces

2 ribs celery, sliced

1 cup corn kernels

2 tablespoons almond butter

2 medium tomatoes, chopped

Direction

1. Heat 1 tablespoon of water in a large soup pot over medium-high heat until it sputters.

2. Cook the onion for 2 minutes, adding a little more water as needed.

3. Add the garlic, Italian seasoning, cumin, and eggplant and stir-fry for 2 to 3 minutes, adding a little more water as needed.

4. Add the carrot, green beans, celery, corn kernels, and ½ cup of water and stir well. Reduce the heat to medium, cover, and cook for 8 to 10 minutes, stirring occasionally, or until the vegetables are tender.

5. Meanwhile, in a bowl, stir together the almond butter and ½ cup of water.

6. Remove the vegetables from the heat and stir in the almond butter mixture and chopped tomatoes. Cool for a few minutes before serving.

Per Serving

Calories: 176 | fat: 5.5g | protein: 5.8g | carbs: 25.4g | fiber: 8.6g | sodium: 198mg

Honey-Glazed Baby Carrots

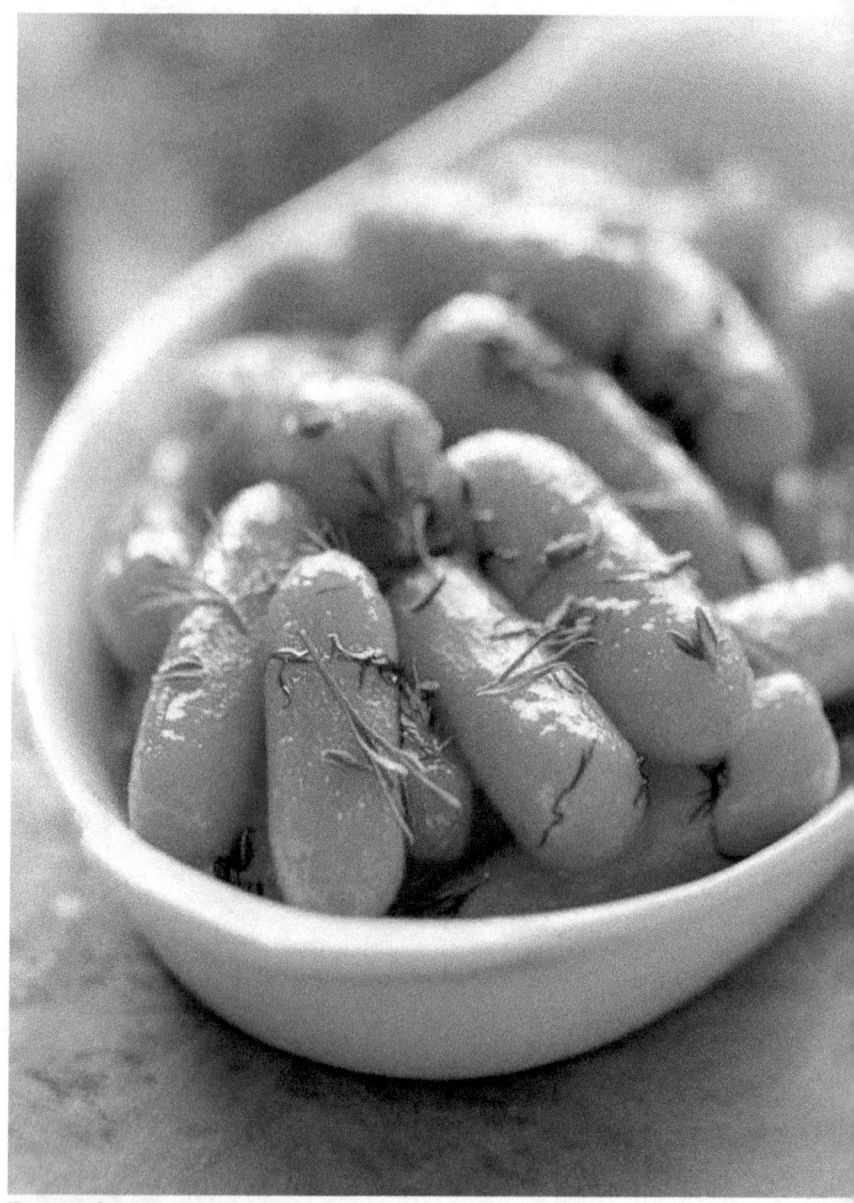

Prep time:

5 minutes | Cook time: 6 minutes | Serves 2

Ingredients

⅔ cup water

1½ pounds (680 g) baby carrots

4 tablespoons almond butter

½ cup honey

1 teaspoon dried thyme

1½ teaspoons dried dill Salt, to taste

Direction

1. Pour the water into the Instant Pot and add a steamer basket. Place t baby carrots in the basket.
2. Secure the lid. Select the Manual mode and set the cooking time for minutes at High Pressure.
3. Once cooking is complete, do a quick pressure release? Carefully op the lid.
4. Transfer the carrots to a plate and set aside.
5. Pour the water out of the Instant Pot and dry it.
6. Press the Sauté button on the Instant Pot and heat the almond butter.
7. Stir in the honey, thyme, and dill.
8. Return the carrots to the Instant Pot and stir until well coated. Sauté f another 1 minute.
9. Taste and season with salt as needed. Serve warm.

Per Serving

Calories: 575 | fat: 23.5g | protein: 2.8g | carbs: 90.6g | fiber: 10.3g | sodiu 547mg

Quick Steamed Broccoli

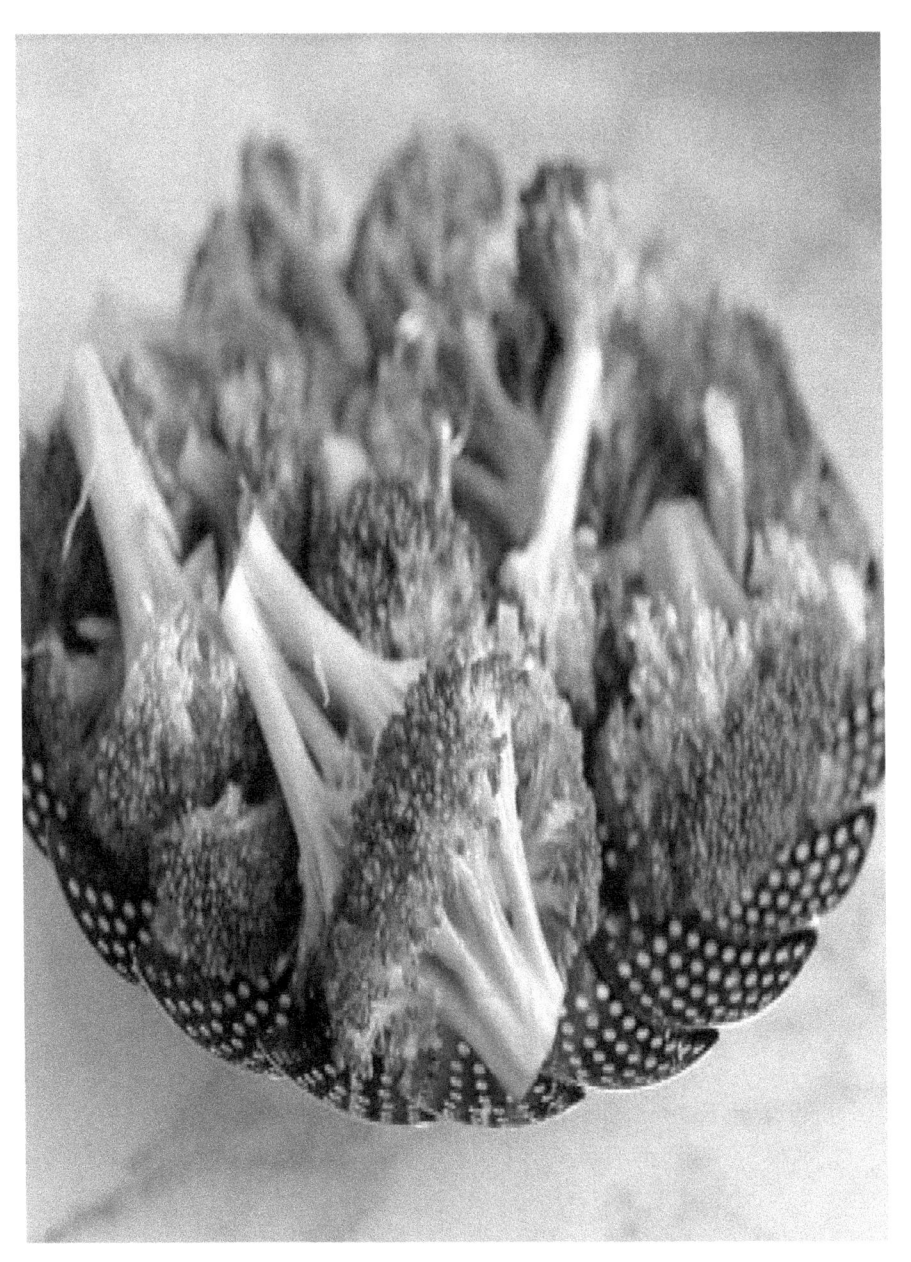

Prep time:
5 minutes | Cook time: 0 minutes | Serves 2

Ingredients

¼ cup water

3 cups broccoli florets

Salt and ground black pepper, to taste

Direction

1. Pour the water into the Instant Pot and insert a steamer basket. Place the broccoli florets in the basket.
2. Secure the lid. Select the Manual mode and set the cooking time for 0 minutes at High Pressure.
3. Once cooking is complete, do a quick pressure release. Carefully open the lid.
4. Transfer the broccoli florets to a bowl with cold water to keep bright green color.
5. Season the broccoli with salt and pepper to taste, then serve.

Per Serving

Calories: 16 | fat: 0.2g | protein: 1.9g | carbs: 1.7g | fiber: 1.6g | sodium: 292mg

Garlic-Butter Asparagus with Parmesan

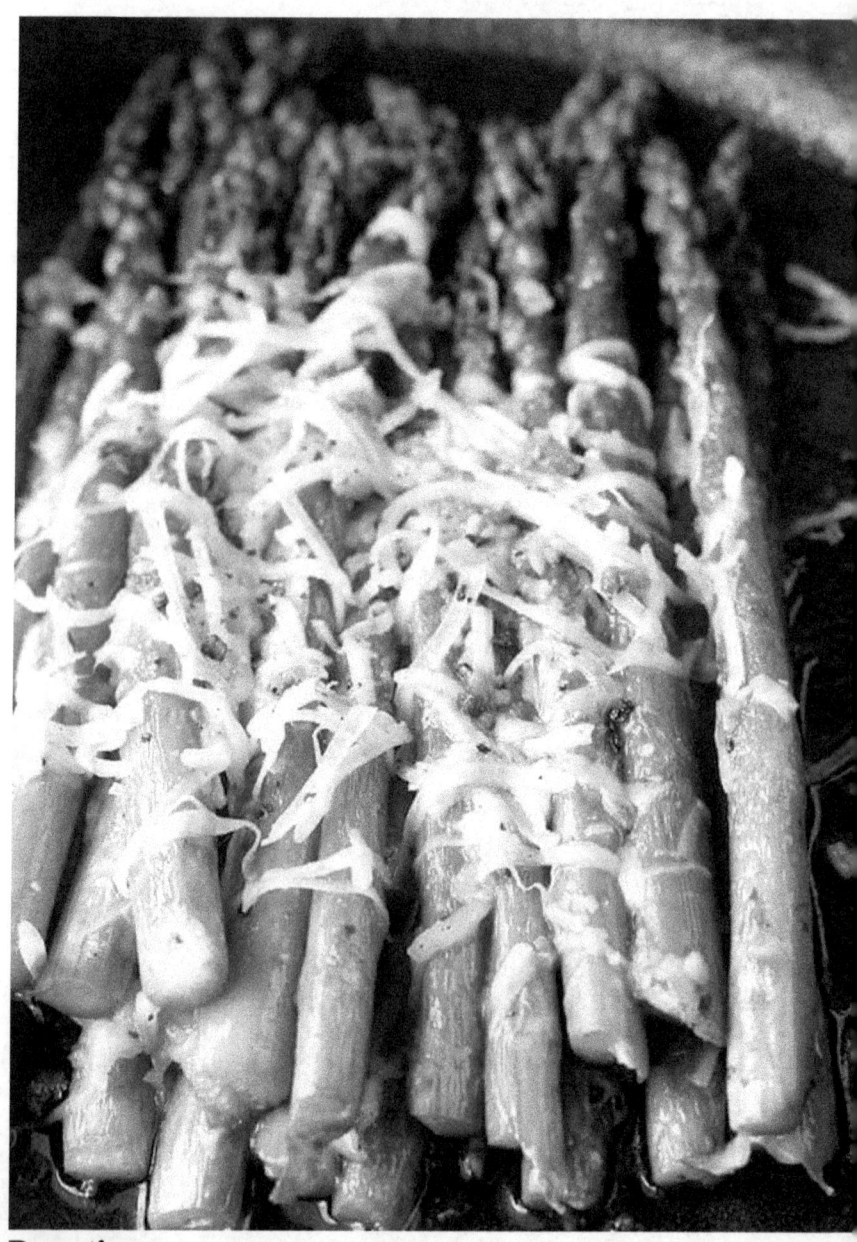

Prep time:

5 minutes | Cook time: 8 minutes | Serves 2

Ingredients

1 cup water

1 pound (454 g) asparagus, trimmed

2 cloves garlic, chopped

3 tablespoons almond butter

Salt and ground black pepper, to taste

3 tablespoons grated Parmesan cheese

Direction

1. Pour the water into the Instant Pot and insert a trivet.
2. Put the asparagus on a tin foil add the butter and garlic. Season to ta with salt and pepper.
3. Fold over the foil and seal the asparagus inside so the foil doesn't cor open. Arrange the asparagus on the trivet.
4. Secure the lid. Select the Manual mode and set the cooking time fo minutes at High Pressure.
5. Once cooking is complete, do a quick pressure release. Carefully op the lid.
6. Unwrap the foil packet and serve sprinkled with the Parmesan cheese

Per Serving

Calories: 243 | fat: 15.7g | protein: 12.3g | carbs: 15.3g | fiber: 7.3g | sodiu 435mg

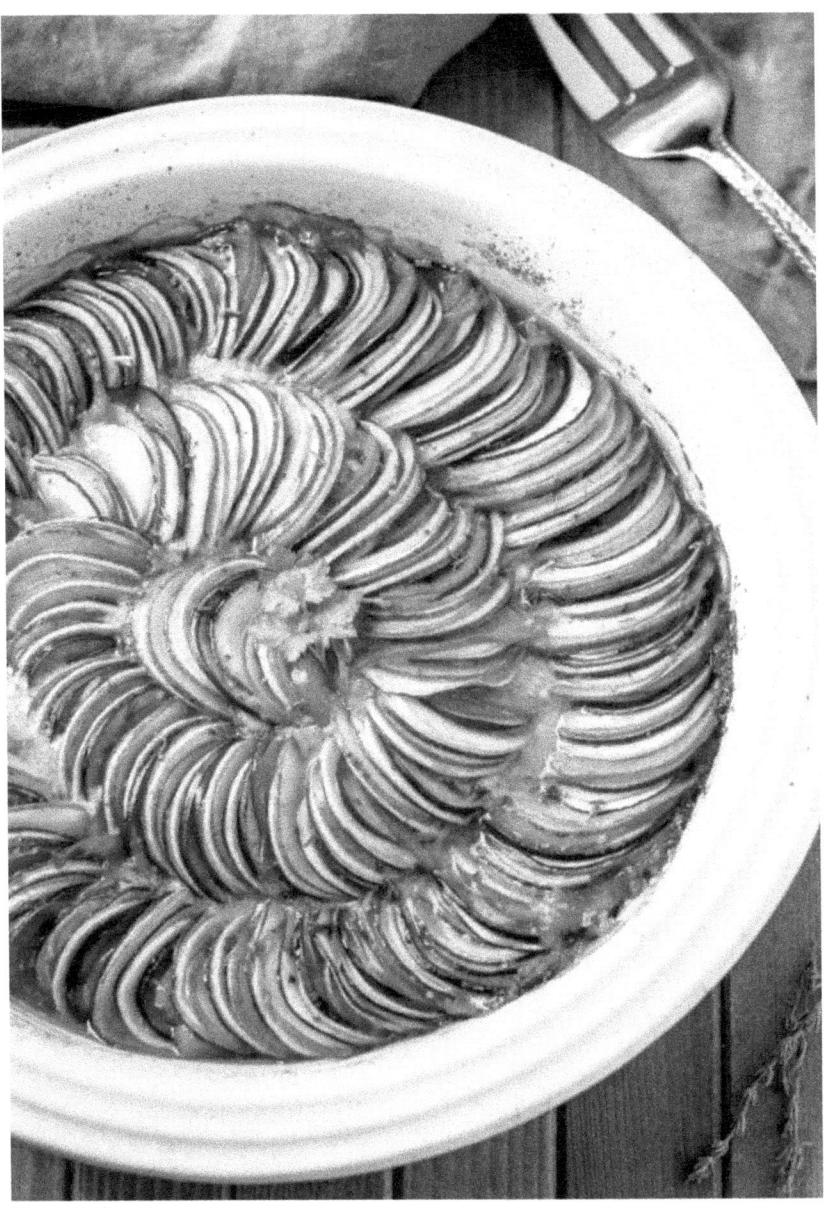

Ratatouille

Prep time:
10 minutes | Cook time: 6 minutes | Serves 4

Ingredients

2 large zucchinis, sliced

2 medium eggplants, sliced

4 medium tomatoes, sliced

2 small red onions, sliced

4 cloves garlic, chopped

2 tablespoons thyme leaves

2 teaspoons sea salt

1 teaspoon black pepper

2 tablespoons balsamic vinegar

4 tablespoons olive oil

2 cups water

Direction

1. Line a springform pan with foil and place the chopped garlic in the bottom.
2. Now arrange the vegetable slices, alternately, in circles.
3. Sprinkle the thyme, pepper and salt over the vegetables. Top with oil and vinegar.
4. Pour a cup of water into the instant pot and place the trivet inside.
5. Secure the lid and cook on Manual function for 6 minutes at High Pressure.
6. Release the pressure naturally and remove the lid.
7. Remove the vegetables along with the tin foil.
8. Serve on a platter and enjoy.

Per Serving

Calories: 240 | fat: 14.3g | protein: 4.7g | carbs: 27.5g | fiber: 10.8g | sodium: 1181mg

Mushroom and Potato Teriyaki

Prep time:

10 minutes | Cook time: 18 minutes | Serves 4

Ingredients

¾ large yellow or white onion, chopped

1½ medium carrots, diced

1½ ribs celery, chopped

1 medium portabella mushroom, diced

¾ tablespoon garlic, chopped

2 cups water

1 pound (454 g) white potatoes, peeled and diced

¼ cup tomato paste

½ tablespoon sesame oil

2 teaspoons sesame seeds

½ tablespoon paprika

1 teaspoon fresh rosemary

¾ cups peas

¼ cup fresh parsley for garnishing, chopped

Direction

1. Add the oil, sesame seeds, and all the vegetables in the instant pot and Sauté for 5 minutes.
2. Stir in the remaining Ingredients and secure the lid.
3. Cook on Manual function for 13 minutes at High Pressure.
4. After the beep, natural release the pressure and remove the lid.
5. Garnish with fresh parsley and serve hot.

Per Serving

Calories: 160 | fat: 3.0g | protein: 4.7g | carbs: 30.6g | fiber: 5.5g | sodium: 52mg

Peanut and Coconut Stuffed Eggplants

Prep time:

15 minutes | Cook time: 9 minutes | Serves 4

Ingredients

1 tablespoon coriander seeds

½ teaspoon cumin seeds

½ teaspoon mustard seeds

2 to 3 tablespoons chickpea flour

2 tablespoons chopped peanuts

2 tablespoons coconut shreds

1-inch ginger, chopped

2 cloves garlic, chopped

1 hot green chili, chopped

½ teaspoon ground cardamom

A pinch of cinnamon

⅓ to ½ teaspoon cayenne

½ teaspoon turmeric

½ teaspoon raw sugar

½ to ¾ teaspoon salt

1 teaspoon lemon juice

Water as needed

4 baby eggplants

Fresh Cilantro for garnishing

Direction

1. Add the coriander, mustard seeds and cumin in the instant pot.
2. Roast on Sauté function for 2 minutes.
3. Add the chickpea flour, nuts and coconut shred to the pot, and roast for 2 minutes.
4. Blend this mixture in a blender, then transfer to a medium-sized bowl.
5. Roughly blend the ginger, garlic, raw sugar, chili, and all the spices in a blender.
6. Add the water and lemon juice to make a paste. Combine it with the dry flour mixture.
7. Cut the eggplants from one side and stuff with the spice mixture.
8. Add 1 cup of water to the instant pot and place the stuffed eggplants inside.
9. Sprinkle some salt on top and secure the lid.
10. Cook on Manual for 5 minutes at High Pressure, then quick release the steam.
11. Remove the lid and garnish with fresh cilantro, then serve hot.

Per Serving

Calories: 207 | fat: 4.9g | protein: 7.9g | carbs: 39.6g | fiber: 18.3g | sodium: 315mg

Cauliflower with Sweet Potato

Prep time:

15 minutes | Cook time: 8 minutes | Serves 8

Ingredients

1 small onion

4 tomatoes

4 garlic cloves, chopped

2-inch ginger, chopped

2 teaspoons olive oil

1 teaspoon turmeric

2 teaspoons ground cumin Salt, to taste

1 teaspoon paprika

2 medium sweet potatoes, cubed small

2 small cauliflowers, diced

2 tablespoons fresh cilantro for topping, chopped

Direction

1. Blend the tomatoes, garlic, ginger and onion in a blender.
2. Add the oil and cumin in the instant pot and Sauté for 1 minute.
3. Stir in the blended mixture and the remaining spices.
4. Add the sweet potatoes and cook for 5 minutes on Sauté
5. Add the cauliflower chunks and secure the lid.
6. Cook on Manual for 2 minutes at High Pressure.
7. Once done, Quick release the pressure and remove the lid.
8. Stir and serve with cilantro on top.

Per Serving

Calories: 76 | fat: 1.6g | protein: 2.7g | carbs: 14.4g | fiber: 3.4g | sodium: 55mg

Potato Curry

Prep time:

10 minutes | Cook time: 30 minutes | Serves 2

Ingredients

2 large potatoes, peeled and diced

1 small onion, peeled and diced

8 ounces (227 g) fresh tomatoes

1 tablespoon olive oil

1 cup water

2 tablespoons garlic cloves, grated

½ tablespoon rosemary

½ tablespoon cayenne pepper

1½ tablespoons thyme

Salt and pepper, to taste

Direction

1. Pour a cup of water into the instant pot and place the steamer trivet inside.
2. Place the potatoes and half the garlic over the trivet and sprinkle some salt and pepper on top.
3. Secure the lid and cook on Steam function for 20 minutes.
4. After the beep, natural release the pressure and remove the lid.
5. Put the potatoes to one side and empty the pot.
6. Add the remaining Ingredients to the cooker and Sauté for 10 minutes.
7. Use an immerse blender to purée the cooked mixture.
8. Stir in the steamed potatoes and serve hot.

Per Serving

Calories: 398 | fat: 7.6g | protein: 9.6g | carbs: 76.2g | fiber: 10.9g | sodium: 111mg

Mushroom, Potato, and Green Bean Mix

Prep time:

10 minutes | Cook time: 18 minutes | Serves 3

Ingredients

1 tablespoon olive oil

½ carrot, peeled and minced

½ celery stalk, minced

½ small onion, minced

1 garlic clove, minced

½ teaspoon dried sage, crushed

½ teaspoon dried rosemary, crushed

4 ounces (113 g) fresh Portabella mushrooms, sliced

4 ounces (113 g) fresh white mushrooms, sliced

¼ cup red wine

1 Yukon Gold potato, peeled and diced

¾ cup fresh green beans, trimmed and chopped

1 cup tomatoes, chopped

½ cup tomato paste

½ tablespoon balsamic vinegar

3 cups water

Salt and freshly ground black pepper to taste

2 ounces (57 g) frozen peas

½ lemon juice

2 tablespoons fresh cilantro for garnishing, chopped

Direction

1. Put the oil, onion, tomatoes and celery into the instant pot and Sauté for 5 minutes.

2. Stir in the herbs and garlic and cook for 1 minute.

3. Add the mushrooms and sauté for 5 minutes. Stir in the wine and cook for a further 2 minutes

4. Add the diced potatoes and mix. Cover the pot with a lid and let the potatoes cook for 2-3 minutes.

5. Now add the green beans, carrots, tomato paste, peas, salt, pepper, water and vinegar.

6. Secure the lid and cook on Manual function for 8 minutes at High Pressure with the pressure valve in the sealing position.

7. Do a Quick release and open the pot, stir the veggies and then add lemon juice and cilantro, then serve with rice or any other of your choice.

Per Serving

Calories: 238 | fat: 5.4g | protein: 8.3g | carbs: 42.7g | fiber: 8.5g | sodium: 113mg

Mushroom Tacos

Prep time:
10 minutes | Cook time: 13 minutes | Serves 3

Ingredients
4 large guajillo chilies

2 teaspoons oil

2 bay leaves

2 large onions, sliced

2 garlic cloves

2 chipotle chillies in adobo sauce

2 teaspoons ground cumin

1 teaspoon dried oregano

1 teaspoon smoked hot paprika

½ teaspoon ground cinnamon, Salt, to taste

¾ cup vegetable broth

1 teaspoon apple cider vinegar

3 teaspoons lime juice

¼ teaspoon sugar

8 ounces (227 g) mushrooms chopped

Whole-wheat tacos, for serving

Direction

1. Put the oil, onion, garlic, salt and bay leaves into the instant pot and Sauté for 5 minutes.
2. Blend the half of this mixture, in a blender, with all the spices and chillies.
3. Add the mushrooms to the remaining onions and Sauté for 3 minutes.
4. Pour the blended mixture into the pot and secure the lid.
5. Cook on Manual function for 5 minutes at High Pressure.
6. Once done, Quick release the pressure and remove the lid.
7. Stir well and serve with tacos.

Per Serving

Calories: 138 | fat: 4.1g | protein: 5.7g | carbs: 23.8g | fiber: 4.8g | sodium: 208mg

Lentils and Eggplant Curry

Prep time:
10 minutes | Cook time: 22 minutes | Serves 4

Ingredients
¾ cup lentils, soaked and rinsed

1 teaspoon olive oil

½ onion, chopped

4 garlic cloves, chopped

1 teaspoon ginger, chopped

1 hot green chili, chopped

¼ teaspoon turmeric

½ teaspoon ground cumin

2 tomatoes, chopped

1 cup eggplant, chopped

1 cup sweet potatoes, cubed

¾ teaspoon salt

2 cups water

1 cup baby spinach leaves

Cayenne and lemon/lime to taste

Pepper flakes (garnish)

Direction

1. Add the oil, garlic, ginger, chili and salt into the instant pot and Sauté for 3 minutes.
2. Stir in the tomatoes and all the spices. Cook for 5 minutes.
3. Add all the remaining Ingredients, except the spinach leaves and garnish.
4. Secure the lid and cook on Manual function for 12 minutes at High Pressure.
5. After the beep, release the pressure naturally and remove the lid.
6. Stir in the spinach leaves and let the pot simmer for 2 minutes on Sauté.
7. Garnish with the pepper flakes and serve warm.

Per Serving

Calories: 88 | fat: 1.5g | protein: 3.4g | carbs: 17.4g | fiber: 3.3g | sodium: 470mg

Sweet Potato and Tomato Curry

Prep time:
5 minutes | Cook time: 8 minutes | Serves 8

Ingredients
2 large brown onions, finely diced

4 tablespoons olive oil

4 teaspoons salt

4 large garlic cloves, diced

1 red chili, sliced

4 tablespoons cilantro, chopped

4 teaspoons ground cumin

2 teaspoons ground coriander

2 teaspoons paprika

2 pounds (907 g) sweet potato, diced

4 cups chopped, tinned tomatoes

2 cups water

2 cups vegetable stock

Lemon juice and cilantro (garnish)

Direction

1. Put the oil and onions into the instant pot and Sauté for 5 minutes.
2. Stir in the remaining Ingredients and secure the lid.
3. Cook on Manual function for 3 minutes at High Pressure.
4. Once done, Quick release the pressure and remove the lid.
5. Garnish with cilantro and lemon juice.
6. Serve.

Per Serving

Calories: 224 | fat: 8.0g | protein: 4.6g | carbs: 35.9g | fiber: 7.5g | sodium: 1385mg

Veggie Chili

Prep time:
15 minutes | Cook time: 10 minutes | Serves 3

Ingredients
½ tablespoon olive oil

1 small yellow onion, chopped

4 garlic cloves, minced

¾ (15-ounce / 425-g) can diced tomatoes

1 ounce (28 g) sugar-free tomato paste

½ (4-ounce / 113-g) can green chilies with liquid

1 tablespoon Worcestershire sauce

2 tablespoons red chili powder

½ cup carrots, diced

½ cup scallions, chopped

½ cup green bell pepper, chopped

¼ cup peas

1 tablespoon ground cumin

½ tablespoon dried oregano, crushed

Salt and freshly ground black pepper to taste

Direction

1. Add the oil, onion, and garlic into the instant pot and Sauté for 5 minutes.
2. Stir in the remaining vegetables and stir-fry for 3 minutes.
3. Add the remaining Ingredients and secure the lid.
4. Cook on Manual function for 2 minutes at High Pressure.
5. After the beep, natural release the pressure and remove the lid.
6. Stir well and serve warm.

Per Serving

Calories: 106 | fat: 3.9g | protein: 3.4g | carbs: 18.0g | fiber: 6.2g | sodium: 492mg

Cabbage Stuffed Acorn Squash

Prep time:

15 minutes | Cook time: 23 minutes | Serves 4

Ingredients

½ tablespoon olive oil

2 medium Acorn squashes

¼ small yellow onion, chopped

1 jalapeño pepper, chopped

½ cup green onions, chopped

½ cup carrots, chopped

¼ cup cabbage, chopped

1 garlic clove, minced

½ (6-ounce / 170-g) can sugar-free tomato sauce

½ tablespoon chili powder

½ tablespoon ground cumin

Salt and freshly ground black pepper to taste

2 cups water

¼ cup Cheddar cheese, shredded

Direction

1. Pour the water into the instant pot and place the trivet inside.
2. Slice the squash into 2 halves and remove the seeds.
3. Place over the trivet, skin side down, and sprinkle some salt and pepper over it.
4. Secure the lid and cook on Manual for 15 minutes at High Pressure.
5. Release the pressure naturally and remove the lid. Empty the pot into a bowl.
6. Now add the oil, onion, and garlic in the instant pot and Sauté for 5 minutes.
7. Stir in the remaining vegetables and stir-fry for 3 minutes.
8. Add the remaining Ingredients and secure the lid.
9. Cook on Manual function for 2 minutes at High Pressure.
10. After the beep, natural release the pressure and remove the lid.
11. Stuff the squashes with the prepared mixture and serve warm.

Per Serving

Calories: 163 | fat: 5.1g | protein: 4.8g | carbs: 28.4g | fiber: 4.9g | sodium: 146mg

Creamy Potato Curry

Prep time:
10 minutes | Cook time: 18 minutes | Serves 4

Ingredients

¾ large yellow or white onion, chopped

1½ ribs celery, chopped

¼ cup carrots, diced

¼ cup green onions

½ cup coconut milk

¾ tablespoon garlic, chopped

1½ cups water

1 pound (454 g) white potatoes, peeled and diced

¼ cup heavy cream

¼ teaspoon thyme

¼ teaspoon rosemary

½ tablespoon black pepper

¾ cup peas Salt, to taste

2 tablespoons fresh cilantro for garnishing, chopped

Direction

1. Add the oil and all the vegetables in the instant pot and Sauté for 5 minutes.
2. Stir in the remaining Ingredients and secure the lid.
3. Cook on Manual function for 13 minutes at High Pressure.
4. Once it beeps, natural release the pressure and remove the lid.
5. Garnish with fresh cilantro and serve hot.

Per Serving

Calories: 210 | fat: 10.1g | protein: 4.1g | carbs: 27.6g | fiber: 4.7g | sodium: 74mg

Mushroom and Spinach Stuffed Peppers

Prep time:

15 minutes | Cook time: 8 minutes | Serves 7

Ingredients

7 mini sweet peppers

1 cup button mushrooms, minced

5 ounces (142 g) organic baby spinach

½ teaspoon fresh garlic

½ teaspoon coarse sea salt

¼ teaspoon cracked mixed pepper

2 tablespoons water

1 tablespoon olive oil

Organic Mozzarella cheese, diced

Direction

1. Put the sweet peppers and water in the instant pot and Sauté for 2 minutes.
2. Remove the peppers and put the olive oil into the pot.
3. Stir in the mushrooms, garlic, spices and spinach.
4. Cook on Sauté until the mixture is dry.
5. Stuff each sweet pepper with the cheese and spinach mixture.
6. Bake the stuffed peppers in an oven for 6 minutes at 400°F (205°C).
7. Once done, serve hot.

Per Serving

Calories: 81 | fat: 2.4g | protein: 4.1g | carbs: 13.2g | fiber: 2.4g | sodium: 217mg

Black Bean and Corn Tortilla Bowls

Prep time:
10 minutes | Cook time: 8 minutes | Serves 4

Ingredients

1½ cups vegetable broth

½ cup tomatoes, undrained diced

1 small onion, diced

2 garlic cloves, finely minced

1 teaspoon chili powder

1 teaspoon cumin

½ teaspoon paprika

½ teaspoon ground coriander

Salt and pepper to taste

½ cup carrots, diced

2 small potatoes, cubed

½ cup bell pepper, chopped

½ can black beans, drained and rinsed

1 cup frozen corn kernels

½ tablespoon lime juice

2 tablespoons cilantro for topping, chopped

Whole-wheat tortilla chips

Direction

1. Add the oil and all the vegetables into the instant pot and Sauté for 3 minutes.
2. Add all the spices, corn, lime juice, and broth, along with the beans, to the pot.
3. Seal the lid and cook on Manual setting at High Pressure for 5 minutes.
4. Once done, natural release the pressure when the timer goes off. Remove the lid.
5. To serve, put the prepared mixture into a bowl.
6. Top with tortilla chips and fresh cilantro.
7. Serve.

Per Serving

Calories: 183 | fat: 0.9g | protein: 7.1g | carbs: 39.8g | fiber: 8.3g | sodium: 387mg

Cauliflower and Broccoli Bowls

Prep time:

5 minutes | Cook time: 7 minutes | Serves 3

Ingredients

½ medium onion, diced

2 teaspoons olive oil

1 garlic clove, minced

½ cup tomato paste

½ pound (227 g) frozen cauliflower

½ pound (227 g) broccoli florets

½ cup vegetable broth

½ teaspoon paprika

¼ teaspoon dried thyme

2 pinches sea salt

Direction

1. Add the oil, onion and garlic into the instant pot and Sauté for 2 minutes.
2. Add the broth, tomato paste, cauliflower, broccoli, and all the spices, to the pot.
3. Secure the lid. Cook on the Manual setting at with pressure for 5 minutes.
4. After the beep, Quick release the pressure and remove the lid.
5. Stir well and serve hot.

Per Serving

Calories: 109 | fat: 3.8g | protein: 6.1g | carbs: 16.7g | fiber: 6.1g | sodium: 265mg

Radish and Cabbage Congee

Prep time:

5 minutes | Cook time: 20 minutes | Serves 3

Ingredients

1 cup carrots, diced

½ cup radish, diced

6 cups vegetable broth

Salt, to taste

1½ cups short grain rice, rinsed

1 tablespoon grated fresh ginger

4 cups cabbage, shredded

Green onions for garnishing, chopped

Direction

1. Add all the Ingredients, except the cabbage and green onions, into the instant pot.
2. Select the Porridge function and cook on the default time and settings.
3. After the beep, Quick release the pressure and remove the lid
4. Stir in the shredded cabbage and cover with the lid.
5. Serve after 10 minutes with chopped green onions on top.

Per Serving

Calories: 438 | fat: 0.8g | protein: 8.7g | carbs: 98.4g | fiber: 6.7g | sodium: 1218mg

Potato and Broccoli Medley

Prep time:
10 minutes | Cook time: 20 minutes | Serves 3

Ingredients
1 tablespoon olive oil

½ white onion, diced

1½ cloves garlic, finely chopped

1 pound (454 g) potatoes, cut into chunks

1 pound (454 g) broccoli florets, diced

1 pound (454 g) baby carrots, cut in half

¼ cup vegetable broth

½ teaspoon Italian seasoning

½ teaspoon Spike original seasoning

Fresh parsley for garnishing

Direction

1. Put the oil and onion into the instant pot and Sauté for 5 minutes.
2. Stir in the carrots, and garlic and stir-fry for 5 minutes.
3. Add the remaining Ingredients and secure the lid.
4. Cook on the Manual function for 10 minutes at High Pressure.
5. After the beep, Quick release the pressure and remove the lid.
6. Stir gently and garnish with fresh parsley, then serve.

Per Serving

Calories: 256 | fat: 5.6g | protein: 9.1g | carbs: 46.1g | fiber: 12.2g | sodium: 274mg

Alphabetical Index

A
Alphabetical Index.. 1

B
Beef and Bean Stuffed Pasta Shells...
Black Bean and Corn Tortilla Bowls..

C
Cabbage Stuffed Acorn Squash..
Caprese Fusilli..
Carrot Risoni..
Cauliflower and Broccoli Bowls..
Cauliflower with Sweet Potato...
Chard and Mushroom Risotto..
Cheesy Sweet Potato Burgers..
Cheesy Tomato Linguine...
Chicken and Spaghetti Ragù Bolognese.................................... 3
Chickpea Lettuce Wraps with Celery..
Creamy Potato Curry...

E
Eggplant and Zucchini Gratin..

G
Grana Padano Risotto..
Garlic-Butter Asparagus with Parmesan.................................... 6

H
Honey-Glazed Baby Carrots.. 6

L

Lentils and Eggplant Curry 84

M

Mushroom and Potato Teriyaki 72

Mushroom and Spinach Stuffed Peppers 94

Mushroom Tacos 82

Mushroom, Potato, and Green Bean Mix 80

P

Parmesan Squash Linguine 34

Peanut and Coconut Stuffed Eggplants 74

Pesto Arborio Rice and Veggie Bowls 13

Potato and Broccoli Medley 102

Potato Curry 78

Q

Quick Steamed Broccoli 63

R

Radish and Cabbage Congee 100

Ratatouille 69

Red Bean Curry 36

Rice and Bean Stuffed Zucchini 16

Roasted Butternut Squash and Rice 10

S

Stir-Fried Eggplant 57

Stuffed Portobello Mushrooms with Spinach 39

Sweet Potato and Tomato Curry 86

T

Turkey and Bell Pepper Tortiglioni..

V

Veggie Chili...8
Veggie-Stuffed Portabello Mushrooms...5

Z

Zoodles with Walnut Pesto..4